D1152198

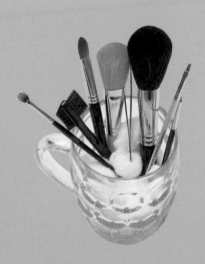

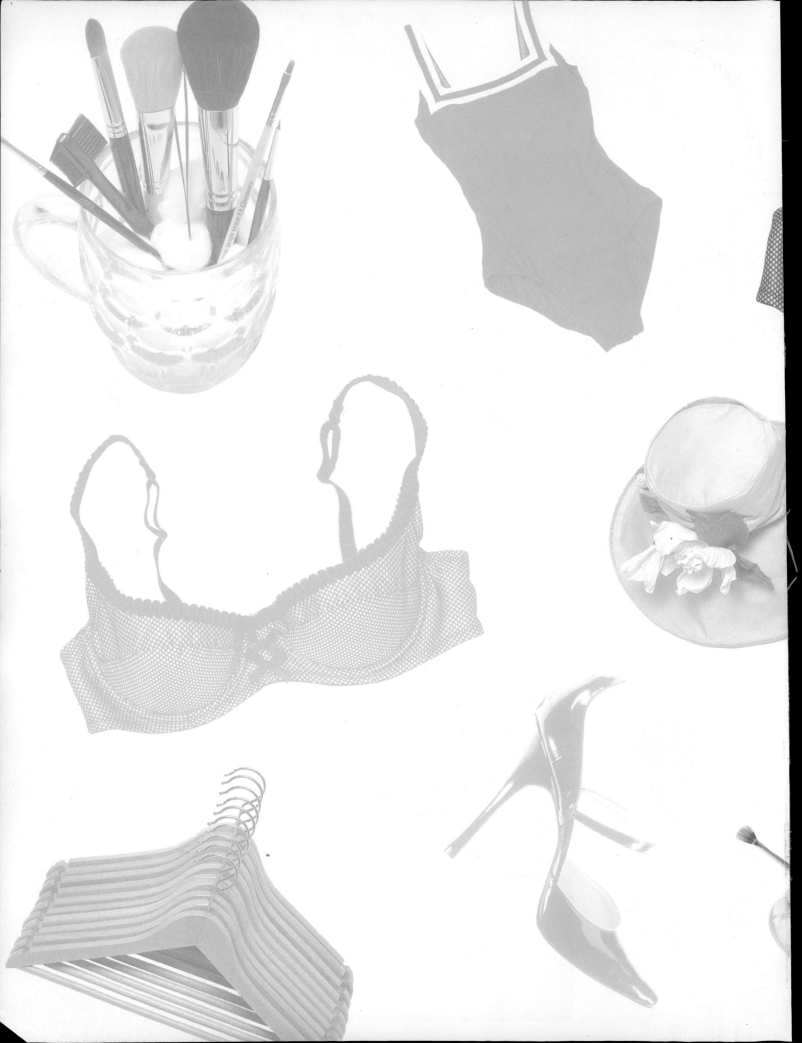

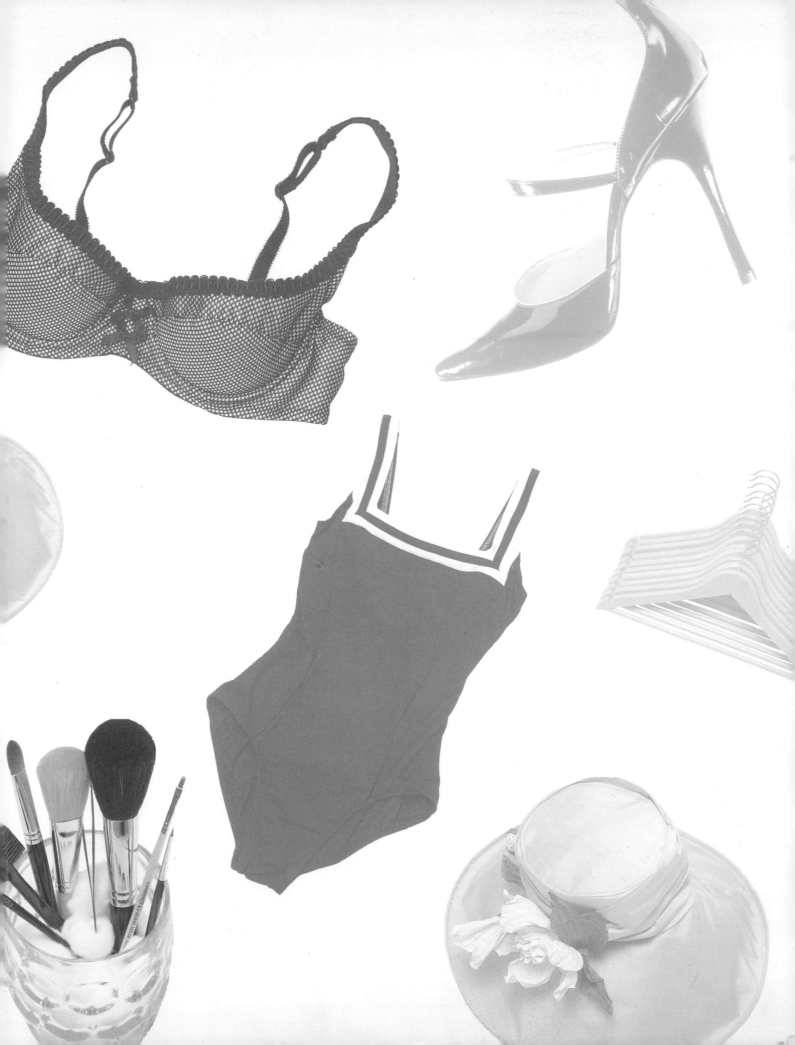

LOOKINGOOD

FASHION AND BEAUTY SOLUTIONS FOR REAL WOMEN

LOOKINGOOD

FASHION AND BEAUTY SOLUTIONS FOR REAL WOMEN

BY

LOWRI TURNER

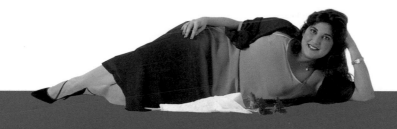

BBC

Contents

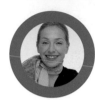
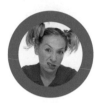
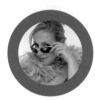
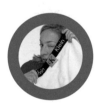
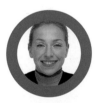
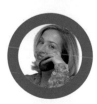
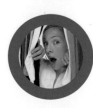

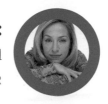
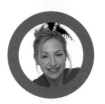
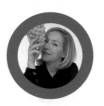
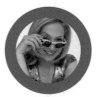
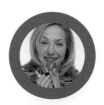
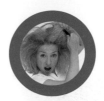

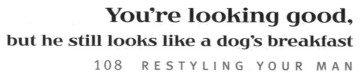

Introduction

When I was first asked if I was interested in getting involved in a new fashion TV programme, I wasn't keen. There were two reasons for my hesitancy. First, I used to be a Fashion Editor. In fact, I was in the fashion business for seven years. But, when you find yourself nodding off to sleep in the middle of an Yves Saint Laurent show, you know you need a career change. So when a chance came to get out of fashion, I did. And, having got out, I wasn't rushing to go back in again.

My second reservation concerned the possible content of the new programme. What the world doesn't need is any more footage of supermodels prancing up and down catwalks in clothes none of the rest of us can afford or get one leg into. That was what I thought when I was told of the planned show and I still think it's true. Pretty pictures of Naomi Campbell and Kate Moss in dresses the size of bath flannels go down a storm with male TV executives, but they don't help Ms Average with the knotty problem of what to put on in the morning.

What changed my mind was that as we – me and the team who would go on to make the first series of *Looking Good* – talked, a clear idea emerged. Real clothes for real women. Rather than featuring designer labels worn by pipe-cleanerthighed models, we'd concentrate on high street clothes and we'd get real women to model them. Women with wobbly bottoms and less-than uplifted bosoms, with fat ankles and upper arms they want to keep covered. Women like you and me.

Regular viewers of *Looking Good* will know that we talk a lot about size on the programme. You will also hear a lot about it in this book. For me, weight is a big issue. I used to tip the scales at 11 stone. I was a size 18. In fact I've been every size between 8 and 18, more than once. Only the panic of seeing my bottom on TV prevents me putting every pound back on again. I may be slim now, but I know the pain of trying to find nice clothes in larger sizes.

I know I'm not alone. Size is the single biggest factor in the fashion-buying behaviour of most women. The size you are dictates what you can buy. The size you want to look determines what you choose to buy. How many times have you stood in a shop changing room and heard someone say, 'Are you sure it's the very latest thing?' Never, right. Instead, all you ever hear is, 'Are you sure it doesn't make me look fat?' Looking thinner is far, far, far more important than looking fashionable to most of us. If we can manage to do both, even better. And that's where this book comes in.

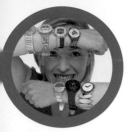

Let's start with a question: hands up who knows exactly what is in their wardrobe – can you describe every garment, its price, provenance and the number of times it has been worn in the last year?

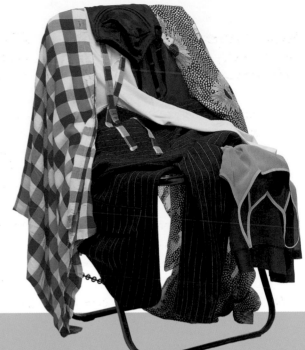

Help! I'm having a fashion emergency

'Did I really buy this?' Sorting out what you've got.

If your fist is waving in the air, then you are either a) a liar or b) a clever Dick or c) suffering from an obsessive compulsive disorder, in which case maybe you'd like to come round to my house and clean my bathroom as I'm sure you'd do a better job than I do.

Most normal women's wardrobes are a mess. Rails are bent under the weight of the mass of garments hung upon them. So tightly packed are these clothes that it is almost impossible to remove one when you want it. And, if you do manage to prise one out, you can't actually wear it because it will need half an hour's ironing just to look halfway presentable. Its hem will be crumpled, its collar will be crushed and the sleeves will be all twisted up.

For every piece of clothing you do succeed in hanging in your wardrobe, there will be half a dozen you don't. These sad specimens spend their lives shoved into carrier bags hidden in some distant corner. When you want to wear one of these, it requires the skill of Doris Stokes to locate it: 'Speak to me blue Top Shop blouse. Did I stick you in the cupboard under the stairs, underneath the broken ironing board and behind the swing ball with the ball missing? Knock once for yes, twice for no.' Invariably, when you do find it, it will be by accident. In the meantime, out of desperation, you will have gone out and bought another one of whatever it was that you were looking for. Now you have two.

You know you need to have a clear-out when...

1

You can no longer shut the doors on a wardrobe or drawers on a chest.

2

Some of your clothes are older than your children.

3

You take the skin off your knuckles trying to get your hand between two items of clothing hanging up in your wardrobe.

4

You have to keep buying duplicates of things you've already got because you can't find them in the mêlée.

5

Everything needs ironing when it comes out of the wardrobe.

In severe cases, furniture has been known to collapse under the strain of containing one woman's wardrobe. Well, my mother's has anyway. So great was (and is) her appetite for clothes that she was forced to buy a cardboard wardrobe to supplement her more conventional wooden ones. This was in the '70s when cardboard was sort of hip. Hip, but not very sturdy. No sooner had she assembled her new cupboard and started to fill it than it began to list. Over time, it gradually took on more and more of the appearance of the leaning wardrobe of Pisa. Finally it toppled over, one side having completely burst open.

It should be pointed out here that the exploding wardrobe incident occurred despite the fact that my mother only ever has half her clothes actually out on display. (The house would probably have exploded if she'd had all of them.) My mother is of the generation who still observe the summer/winter wardrobe ritual. In some cultures they greet the arrival of a new season by slaughtering a small animal. My mother brings down a trunk from the loft.

The summer/winter wardrobe thing

The summer/winter wardrobe thing, though a bit old-fashioned, is actually a very good idea. The basic plan is that twice a year you do a sartorial swapsy. At the beginning of the summer, you pack all your cold-weather clothing in a suitcase and put it away, then get out your summer things and hang them up. When winter arrives, you retrieve the suitcase, take out all your woollies and pack away your summer stuff.

This saves a lot of space, stops you crushing everything and means you don't get bored with your clothes. Plus, it means you have to look at everything you own twice a year, giving you an opportunity to throw out stuff you don't want, or need, or which doesn't fit. That's the theory anyway, though in my mum's case the throwing out bit didn't quite happen.

If you are an absolutely appalling hoarder, then the summer/winter wardrobe ritual may be your only hope. Still, you need to consider a few points first.

Do you have a loft/attic? Packing things into a suitcase is all very well if you've got somewhere to put it. If you live in a studio apartment the size of a rabbit hutch, short of planting the suitcase in the centre of the floor and explaining it away as a post-modern coffee table, you're scuppered.

Do you have an active social life? All that packing and unpacking takes time. Given the choice between a night down the pub getting slaughtered and a night folding sweaters, which would you choose?

Do you have access to a strong man at least twice a year? Depending on how much you're hoarding, that trunk is going to be heavy. You could try dragging it down on your own. It'll be much easier if you have someone with a need to prove his machismo by carrying it for you.

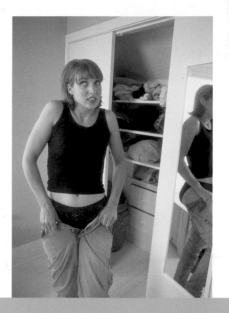

'Perhaps that donut wasn't such a good idea.' If it doesn't fit, throw it out.

Less really is more. Edit your wardrobe.

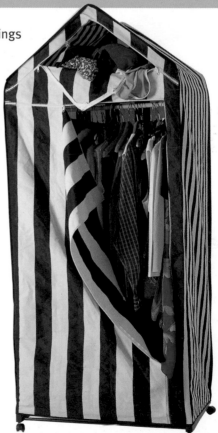

So why do we put ourselves through this?

Men don't understand about women and clothes. 'What do you mean you've got nothing to wear? You've got wardrobes full of clothes,' they say. But a woman's wardrobe is essentially a work in progress. This is because the woman herself is invariably a work in progress. She's trying to lose a stone so she can get into that mini-dress/bikini/pair of size 10 jeans.

This state of limbo is, of course, a huge mistake. Either you never lose that weight, in which case you've wasted an awful lot of money making yourself depressed – every time you open the wardrobe that tiny garment just stares accusingly at you – or you do and you put it all back on again within six months. I myself have three sets of clothes – fat, thin and middling – which I wear according to whether I'm in a Mars Bar ice-cream period or not. When Mars Bar ice-creams first came out I put

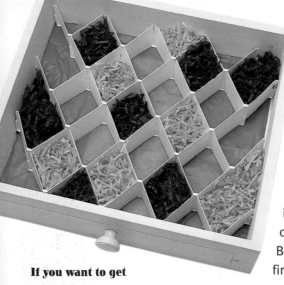

If you want to get really anal, try drawer dividers.

Wood or wire? The choice is yours.

on a stone in a month so addicted to them did I become. I used to go to different shops to buy my supplies so no one shop owner knew how many I was eating and thought I was a complete glutton. These days, I can't even eat one. I know if I do, I'll be back to a family pack a day.

As a result of my yo-yoing weight, I have my three wardrobes down to pat. The fat one is full of tunics and wide trousers and the thin one features a lot of little Lycra tops. It's the middling one I wear most. It has a lot of black in it and, while the trousers are slim-legged, all the jackets are safely bottom covering. So great is the gulf between the fat and thin me, I even have to have underwear in a range of sizes.

Having gone on so much about not hoarding clothes, it might seem strange that I still keep so much stuff I can't wear. But there's an exception to the 'clear out your wardrobe regularly' rule and that exception is those of us whose weight goes up and down. I used to throw the fat stuff out every time I lost weight, but it's bloody expensive to do that – and a real downer too. If it's depressing to put on a stone, how much more depressing is it to have to spend money on a whole new wardrobe to cover the fat bits?

When you have been through everything, you can put the, hopefully, much smaller pile of clothes you're keeping back in your wardrobe. Take the opportunity to

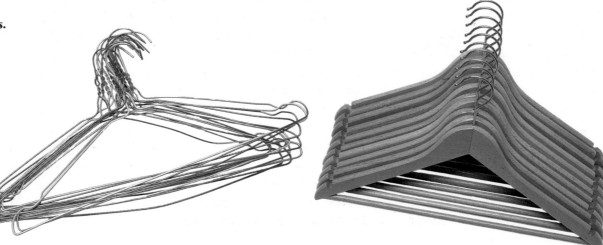

ORGANIZING
WHAT YOU'VE GOT

Whether your weight yo-yos or is stable, you will probably come to a point where you have to sort out what you've got. Set aside an afternoon (it will take you at least that long), clear some floor space and take a deep breath. Be ruthless, but be realistic. Start by sorting all your clothes into three piles:

PILE ONE
The clothes you wear a lot. Take a close look at these. It's amazing how tatty a favourite garment can get without you noticing. If buttons need replacing or a hem is beginning to come down, get out a needle and thread and do it straight away. Don't leave it till later. It'll sit in a pile in the corner of the bathroom and you'll have to step over it every time you want to brush your teeth. The same goes for shoes that need re-soling or heeling. Seize the day.

PILE TWO
This is stuff you haven't worn recently but you think either it might come back into fashion or you spent so much on it that you can't bear to admit defeat and chuck it out. It's this pile that is the most tricky. You need to work out what can be transferred on to pile number one and saved, and what really is past it.

Be honest. If you haven't worn it for six months, you probably aren't going to. On the other hand, maybe the problem is cosmetic. Could a skirt be shortened, the buttons changed on a cardi, or the waist-band on a pair of trousers be loosened? You could be deluding yourself, but if you think there is a way to save something, give it a go.

PILE THREE
These are the things you know you aren't going to wear again. Either they were a mistake in the first place or they are so out of fashion they'll never come back. Everything in this pile goes in a bin bag to the nearest charity shop.

create some sort of system. You don't have to get Howard Hughes about it, but putting all your jackets together, blouses in one place, etc., will make finding things much quicker in the morning. You could go a step further and group clothes by colour as well. It just depends how anal you want to be.

Wood or wire?
On the subject of wood or wire hangers, I'm flexible. Certainly, for anything with a padded shoulder a preformed hanger (wood or plastic) is essential. Otherwise it will look like an old dishrag. But wood hangers take up a lot of rail space and, whatever so-called wardrobe consultants say, if space is limited, I think you're better off putting blouses, shirts and tee-shirts on wire hangers.

If, once you've sorted your clothes out, you find yourself gripped by an organiza-tional evangelical zeal, you could opt for drawer dividers as well. If you've never seen these plastic miracles, let me explain: they unfold into the equivalent of a wine rack for your drawer, only you don't put bottles of wine in the holes, you put in socks and underwear. You can get these dividers from good haberdashers or branches of John Lewis. They make seeing what you've got very easy.

Shoe tidies, be they of the rigid rack type or fabric hanging ones (as famously favoured by Cherie Blair), are another boon. Rather than having to wade through a jum-ble of shoes to find a pair, you can select the ones you want straight away. Plus, they don't get so scuffed. If you don't want to shell out for a shoe tidy, you can always save the boxes your shoes come in. Take a magic marker and write what shoe is inside on the side of every box so you can find the pair you want quickly and easily.

Now you've done the boring bit, it's time for some fun: let's go shopping!

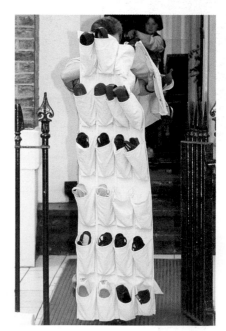

Little Miss Organized. Cherie Blair and her shoes move house.

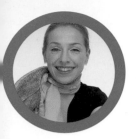

Sorry, did I say shopping was fun? If you're a six-foot supermodel who wears a perfect size 10 and has a bank balance the size of Venezuela's gross national product, then it must be a breeze.

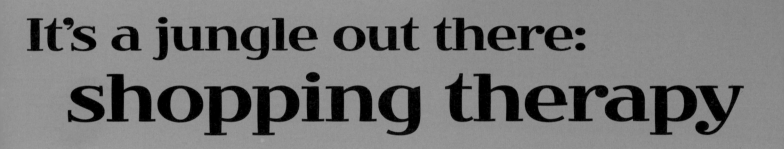

It's a jungle out there:
shopping therapy

You can walk into any designer store you please, pick something off the rack, know it will fit and know you can afford it. Then you hand over your credit card and go off to pick at a salad (no dressing) at a chic pavement eaterie. For mere mortals with budgetary constraints, spare tyre problems and possibly kids to think about, it's more tricky. You try getting a buggy up the steps to Chanel!

Still, whatever problems you may have, you can make shopping a whole lot more enjoyable if you learn how to do it effectively. Effective shopping is about planning; it's about being realistic and not letting your heart rule your head. It's about having a system and sticking to it. I know this all sounds

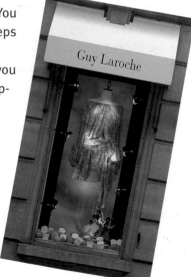

rather dull, but you do have a choice. You can just go with the flow, but if you do that one of two things will happen:

1 You'll come home with carrier bags full of things you realize you hate as soon as you put them on the kitchen table.
2 You won't buy anything at all.

There is something incredibly dispiriting about dragging round the shops and coming away with nothing. I tend to stave off my sense of failure by buying a three-pack of knickers at Marks and Spencer – you get something in a bag and you can never have too many three-packs – but it doesn't really work. It's a bit like going on a big game safari and not catching sight of a single elephant, hippo or tiger. Your camcorder is poised, but all you see is a lonely wildebeest. Wildebeest are fine, but that's not why you came to Africa, is it?

HOW TO SHOP EFFECTIVELY

1 LOOK AT WHAT YOU'VE GOT BEFORE YOU GO SHOPPING **2** ALWAYS BUY THE RIGHT SIZE **3** DON'T BELIEVE SHOP ASSISTANTS **4** TAKE SOMEONE WITH YOU WHOSE OPINION YOU TRUST **5** TRY ON BEFORE YOU BUY **6** REMEMBER THAT A DESIGNER LABEL IS NO GUARANTEE THAT IT'S A NICE GARMENT **7** DON'T BE SEDUCED BY THE SALES INTO BUYING THINGS YOU DON'T WANT, NEED OR LIKE

Buying a new piece of clothing is like embarking on a new relationship. You come to both with a history. You need to examine your pattern of behaviour to see if that new blouse/that new bloke is really right for you. To do this, you need to look at your wardrobe. If it is filled entirely with trousers, you're getting a pretty clear message. It's pointless buying a skirt because you won't wear it. Similarly, if you've bought pink before, but somehow it has lain, unworn, at the back of a drawer, then don't buy it again. You need to learn from your mistakes to shop effectively.

You will by now, of course, have reorganized your wardrobe (cue: mass clearing of throats). OK, you probably haven't. Never mind. Take a long, cool look at what you've got and analyse which things you wear most and why. Then try and buy in the same vein. If there is a black mini that you can hardly bear to send to the dry cleaners because you love it so much, try and purchase a duplicate. I know it doesn't sound very thrilling, but at least you won't make any huge mistakes.

Alternatively, you could opt to plug the gaps in your wardrobe. Maybe you bought a navy jacket and never quite got around to buying any navy trousers to go with it. Or, perhaps you have a dress that needs a particular style of high heel and you haven't been able to wear it because you have been unable to find that shoe. Go out and get the shoes.

If you are plugging the gaps, remember to take the outfit you're trying to complete with you. Never trust your memory. It plays tricks. This is especially important if you're trying to find a colour match. Yes, it's a pain to have to lug stuff around – you're loaded down before you even begin – but it's essential. It's fatally easy to be just a shade off. Some colours are more difficult than others. There are about a hundred navies and red is also tricky. One more tip: take the piece of clothing and the garment it is supposed to match to somewhere there is natural light. What looks the same under fluorescent light might not be the same in daylight.

Take your time and ask yourself, 'Do I really want/need this, and will it go with anything I've already got?'

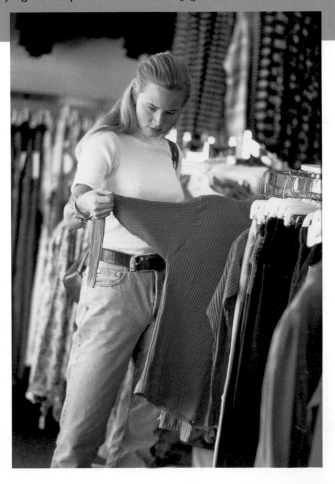

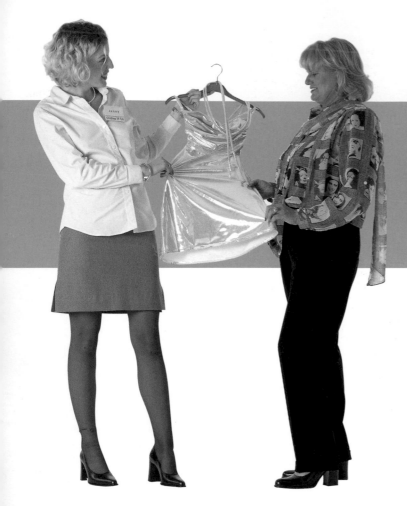

Be honest. It may
be gorgeous, but
if it's the size of a
bath flannel, will
it really suit you?

No, you're not going to lose a stone by Friday

Next you need to know your size. This may sound obvious, but it's amazing how we can hoodwink ourselves into thinking we are still the size we used to be a year, five years, ten years ago. And that doesn't have to mean we're bigger than we think we are either. Anyone who has ever lost a lot of weight will be familiar with phantom fat syndrome. This is where you automatically reach for a size 16 when you're only a 12.

Once you know what size you are, you must buy clothes in that size. Again, this sounds so obvious as to be hardly worth saying. Except, who can put their hand on their heart and say they have never bought anything that they couldn't quite fit into? This is 'it's so lovely I'm sure I can lose enough weight to get into it' syndrome. It's

bad for your wallet and corrosive for your soul. No matter how gorgeous a garment is, if it doesn't fit, it's a waste of money. And thinking it will fit if you lose just a couple of pounds is pointless. If you're that sure you're going to lose the weight, come back and buy the garment when you have done.

Knowing your size is one thing, but what complicates matters is that shops vary so much in their sizing. In the rag trade it's well known that some stores size up their garments, putting a size 12 label on a size 14, say, so as to please their customers. In a fit of euphoria at being able to squeeze into a garment a size smaller than she thought she was, the customer is supposed to reach for her cheque-book and pay whatever price the shop is asking. There is some justification for this belief. There is nothing that makes you want to buy more than thinking you are slimmer than you are.

Stores such as Wallis and Principles are apt to cut on the generous side. 'Middle market' ranges – AKA those aimed at women over 25 – stocked by department stores, Jaeger and Planet for example, also expect their customers to have the occasional square meal. On the other hand, teenage stores such as Kookai, Top Shop and Miss Selfridge are inclined to make things small, very small. So, if you try on a 12 in Kookai and it won't go over your bottom, cheer up, it's them not you.

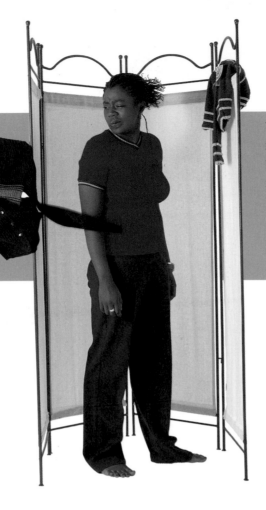

Yes, it's a pain in the bottom, but you must try it on before you buy.

Are you being served? Not likely

The first person you encounter in a shop is the shop assistant. Note that word 'assistant'. He or she is there to assist you. Unfortunately, this is not always the case. That's putting it politely. To be blunter, some shop assistants are completely useless. They are usually too busy discussing last night's date to take any notice of you.

Not all shop assistants are customer unfriendly. There is a sort of hierarchy of awfulness. At the bottom are the staff who work in teen stores. To be fair to them, they're probably paid shirt buttons. Also, since they are invariably teenagers themselves, their hormones are running wild. They'd much rather be out snogging someone called Darren or Shane than serving you.

Only a rung or two up from this level are those snooty assistants employed by swishy designer emporia. Marginally less welcoming than a warder on *Prisoner Cell Block H*, they give the impression they're doing you a favour just by letting you into the shop. Intimidation is the name of their game, but it's an easy one to scupper. The thing to remember here is that while they might look a million dollars in their designer outfit, it probably doesn't belong to them. It's common practice at this level of the market for a shop assistant to select something from the stock first thing in the

morning then put it back again at night. At least you own the clothes you're wearing.

The best shop assistants are to be found in the middle-of-the-road shops, the ones that aren't trying to be too trendy or too upmarket and that aren't horrendously busy. And, if you do find a good shop assistant, make use of them. If you don't see your size on the rack, ask if they've got it in the stock room. If they check and say no, ask them to phone another branch to find out if they've got it there. A good shop assistant shouldn't make you feel you're asking too much. Remember, the customer is always right.

Still, the shop assistant may be good, but there is one thing you should never take from them: advice. Most are on commission. They are biased. They'd say that Waynetta Slob looks like Elle McPherson if they thought it would get them a sale.

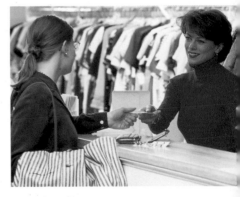

Nice smile, shame about the attitude. Never trust a sales assistant. She speaks with forked tongue.

Trust me, I'm a personal shopper

There is an exception to the 'never trust a sales assistant' rule. Most big department stores now have a Personal Shopping Suite. This is a ritzy little office, tucked away in a corner of one of the sales floors. It usually has three or four changing rooms and a couple of sofas, piles of magazines, and posh twigs in a vase. It's a bit like a very glamorous gynaecologist's office, but without the stirrups.

Anyway, the idea is that you make an appointment and a Personal Shopper then goes through the kind of clothes you're looking for. You tell her your size and give her a budget to work to and then, while you sit on the sofa drinking coffee, she schleps around the store finding things for you to try on. She comes back and you get to try her selection of clothes on in the civilized atmosphere of the Personal Shopping Suite, away from crowds and hassle. Plus, you get her advice.

Amazingly, this service is free and you don't have to buy a certain amount of clothes to get it. In fact, you don't have to buy anything at all. You could spend three hours there and walk away with your cheque-book unopened. Most don't, of course. They spend lots, which is how the stores can provide the service in the first place.

As for the quality of the advice, it depends entirely on the store. If you are close to a large town with more than one department store, go and look at the windows. If they look mumsy, that's how you will look by the time one of their staff has finished with you. If the clothes in the window look stylish, you're on to a safer bet. After all, they can only dress you in their own stock, so if it's any good, the chances are you'll come out looking halfway decent.

Shopping is like drinking: it should never be done alone.

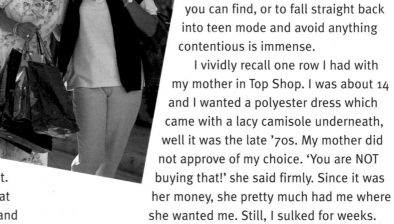

If you don't want to buy all your clothes from one store, or you don't have the chance to use a Personal Shopper, the next best thing is to take someone shopping with you, but who?

Mother knows best?

Taking your mother is one option. This is fine if you're buying jeans or a new duffle coat, not so fine if you fancy a bit of exotic lingerie or a plunge-necked top. To your mum you're always her little girl whose excesses need to be restrained.

Besides, every woman remembers the battles she had with her mum about clothes during her teenage years. The temptation either to get your own back by buying the most outrageous garment you can find, or to fall straight back into teen mode and avoid anything contentious is immense.

I vividly recall one row I had with my mother in Top Shop. I was about 14 and I wanted a polyester dress which came with a lacy camisole underneath, well it was the late '70s. My mother did not approve of my choice. 'You are NOT buying that!' she said firmly. Since it was her money, she pretty much had me where she wanted me. Still, I sulked for weeks. Actually, I'm still sulking.

'But the match is on in five minutes.' Why you should definitely leave HIM at home.

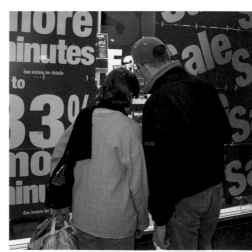

It's very nice, but so was the first one you tried on

Another option is to take your boyfriend/ husband. This is an even more unwise choice. Men fall into two types: those who love shopping and those who loathe it. To take the latter first, he will transmogrify into a fractious toddler the moment you walk into Dorothy Perkins. 'Are we going home yet?' he will say about five minutes after you've arrived. Variations on this theme include, 'There's a McDonalds over the road,' 'The match is starting in five minutes' and 'I promised your dad I'd give him a hand with those shelves.' Anything to get out of having to tramp around shops all afternoon.

You see these shopping refuseniks slumped disconsolately outside shop changing rooms, where they are tripped over by other shoppers. That they find shopping painful would not really matter, but their impatience is apt to affect your decisions. Ask this type of man what he thinks about an outfit and he will start off by saying, 'It's all right'. That's in the first shop. By shop number two it will be: 'It's very nice.' By shop number three he will be bursting with enthusiasm for just about anything you put on. This has absolutely nothing to do with the improving quality of the merchandise and everything to do with the fact that he wants you to buy some- thing, anything, so he can go home, which is where you should have left him in the first place.

The man who loves shopping is scarcely more useful. For a start, he'll slow you down. For him, ladies' shops are Aladdin's caves of unfamiliar treasures. He'll want you to try everything on, even though you know it won't look any good on you. It is very charming when a man thinks you are physically perfect and can therefore look like Cindy Crawford in everything from a pinafore to a leather mini. It is downright

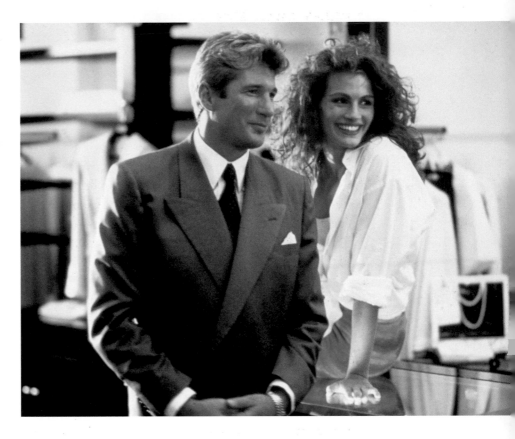

maddening, however, when he refuses to accept that you know better. A woman doesn't become an adult without having worked out what suits her and what doesn't. And, no man is ever going to fully appreciate the need to cover certain bits – tops of arms, whole of bottom. This takes time to explain. Leave him at home too.

The best person to take shopping with you is a girlfriend. Not just any girlfriend, though. I can remember going to try on *Grease*-style stretch satin jeans with a couple of girlfriends after school. They were tall and slim. I was not. As they admired their flat stomachs encased in shiny turquoise Spandex, I was in the corner cringing because I couldn't get the trousers over my thighs. The lesson to be learned? Never go shopping with a girlfriend more than two sizes slim- mer than you.

He likes shopping and he picks up the tab? Only in the movies.

Changing room torture

This story also introduces another sore point of mine: changing rooms. They have improved since the days when entering one was like going below decks on a slave ship. Today, only the naffest store has a communal changing room. Still, the lighting always makes your skin look faintly green, there are never enough hooks and the space is always cramped. If you bend over to put on your shoes, you bottom is apt to pierce the curtain and emerge into the big wide world, somewhat embarrassing if you're wearing only your knickers.

My particular pet hate is changing rooms that don't have mirrors. You have to walk out of your cubicle and prance around in the middle of the shop just so you can see how hideous you look. Why do stores do this? Do they want to humiliate their customers? Apparently so.

Still, however awful changing rooms are, they are a necessary evil. It's tempting to say to yourself that you'll try it on at home and if it doesn't fit you'll bring it back, but how many times have you said that and merely tossed another carrier bag on to the Clothes That Look Horrible mountain that is rapidly growing in one corner of your wardrobe? Now, repeat after me, 'I will not buy anything unless I have tried it on first.'

There is one way to make trying on clothes in shops a slightly less disgusting experience. This involves selecting the right clothes to wear to try on clothes in a changing room. This probably sounds odd. After all, you're only going to take whatever you have off. But, there are good reasons for choosing your outfit carefully.

Don't get hot under the collar. Remember to choose changing-room friendly clothing when going on shopping expeditions.

Psychology

Trying clothes on in a changing room is torture. The light is bad and you feel awful. By the time you've been unable to do the waist up on a couple of pairs of trousers you're going to feel like killing yourself. To bolster yourself against sinking into this depression, you need to feel good about yourself to begin with. Wearing an outfit you like and know you look good in will give you confidence, keep your spirits up and get you more respect from snotty sales girls.

Building this confidence starts before you actually get dressed though. Shave your legs and armpits and, if you're going to be trying on swimwear, do your bikini line as well. If this sounds too much trouble, bear in mind how you'll feel if you do encounter a communal changing room and you've got the Forest of Dean in each armpit.

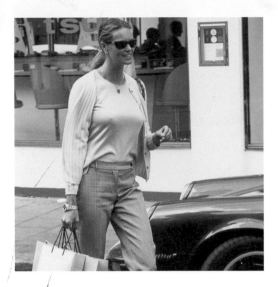

Even celebs have to carry their own bags occasionally.

Also, put on some make-up. Not so much that you'll leave a layer of it on everything you try on, but enough to make you feel that you are vaguely attractive. Again, it'll impress sales girls and they'll give you better service. And make sure you're wearing your best underwear. Remember what your grandma said about wearing clean knickers in case you got knocked down? Well, that goes double for a changing room curtain being opened by a total stranger by mistake. I know – it's happened to me.

Do wear
your best outfit
classy underwear
make-up

Don't wear
grubby jumper and leggings
greying bra and tights with ladders in them

Practicality

You're going to be doing a lot of walking, so wear comfortable shoes. That said, nothing looks worse than a mini skirt with ankle socks and trainers. Take a pair of nice shoes in a bag with you, then you can get a proper idea of how you look in a smart skirt or dress. Also make sure you wear clothes that are quick and easy to get in and out of, or you'll spend more time buttoning yourself up than actually shopping. Very tight clothing or anything made from synthetic fabrics will stick to you and be very unpleasant to peel off and put back on again.

Do wear
tops with loose necks or those that do up with zips
trousers or skirts with elasticated waists
pull-on shoes
natural fibres

Don't wear
polo necks
anything with a lot of buttons or fiddly lacing
tight jeans
synthetic fibres

OK, you've got your girlfriend and your outfit sorted and you've done your bikini line, so what do you buy? Let's start with what not to buy.

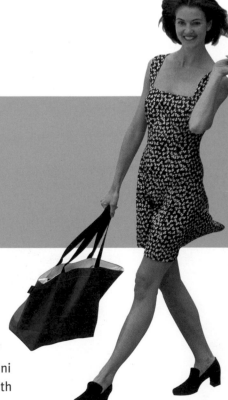

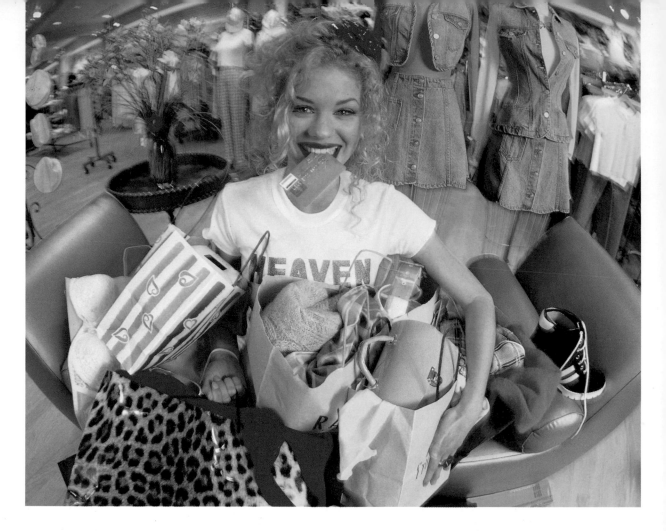

She's gotta have it

How many times have you been on a bus, seen something in a shop window and decided there and then that you've got to have it? You've got off the bus, gone into the shop and before you can say 'next month's credit card bill', you've bought it. To paraphrase the scent ad, 'women can't help acting on impulse'. Well, some women can't anyway.

Stores spend large amounts of money employing camp men to dress windows just so you can't resist what's in them. The problem is what is eye-catching behind a sheet of glass is rarely what you'd call wearable on a day-to-day basis. For eye-catching, you can invariably read impractical and over-priced. I ask you, if you owned a shop and in some fit of lunacy you'd bought a whole load of puce fake fur jackets that you needed to get rid of quick because it was June and the weather reports predicted an imminent heatwave,

Shopping on impulse: buy in haste, feel guilty for ages afterwards.

what would you do? You'd stick them in the window, wouldn't you? Retailers don't necessarily put the best stuff in the window, just the things they want or need to shift a lot of fast.

A factor that can fuel impulse buying is alcohol. You've had a great lunch with a girlfriend, shared a bottle of wine, maybe even a brandy or two afterwards. Then, you decide to do a bit of 'window shopping'. This is when the alarm bells should go off in your head. You are in no state to make sound sartorial judgements. In your inebriated state you'd buy the changing room curtain if they'd sell it to you. Never, ever go shopping when you've had a drink.

If you're a New Age babe, you can add to that: never go shopping after a massage, reflexology session or yoga class. They all leave you lightheaded and in a dangerously good mood. I once had a back massage in a department store beauty salon. Cunningly they'd put the salon right next to some of the most expensive clothes in the shop. Half an hour after my sinews had been pummelled, I found myself trying on £500 jackets. Fortunately, somebody walked past me wearing Dior Poison and that sobered me up fast.

If it says 50% off, it must be good

Sales are another impulse-buying nightmare. All those 50% off banners and 'best buy' stickers can send some women into a trance-like state where they buy anything their hand touches. But, it should be remembered, the reason something is in a sale is that no one wanted to pay full price for it. There is probably a good reason for that. Maybe it fits badly, or is an odd colour. It may be that it is wildly unflattering or so trendy that it's gone out of fashion while it's been on the hanger. Whatever the reason, think very carefully before you shout 'bargain'.

The way sales are organized is also guaranteed to wither your normal judgement. Big scrums of people and large piles of clothes give a jumble sale feel, which is OK if the clothes are genuinely cheap, but not so OK if they come with price tags reading in the hundreds of pounds. Stores deliberately foster this bazaar-type look at sales time because it gives a 'buzzy' atmosphere in which you are more likely to buy.

Then there is the ordeal factor. Shopping on the first day of the sales in particular is unpleasant. It is hot and crowded. In the same way that climbers who have scaled some particularly tricky peak feel an irresistible urge to plant a flag on the top, so you, having endured sales hell, feel you ought to buy something. You feel you deserve to buy something. And so, you buy something. The trouble is, it's not necessarily any use to you.

Talk to a French woman and she'll tell you she avoids sales altogether. She buys at the beginning of the season, when all the new ranges are in so she can have maximum choice, albeit at maximum price. She eschews sales as full of a load of old rubbish. This is perhaps a bit harsh. There are bargains to be had in the sales. Before you buy ask yourself three questions:

1 Would I buy it at full price?
2 Would I be embarrassed taking it to the dry cleaner?
3 Do I have to breathe in to do up the waistband?

If the answer is yes to the first and no to the second and third questions, then go ahead and buy it (if you've got the money). You can always take it back if you decide you hate it and then you get to go shopping all over again.

Now for what to buy...

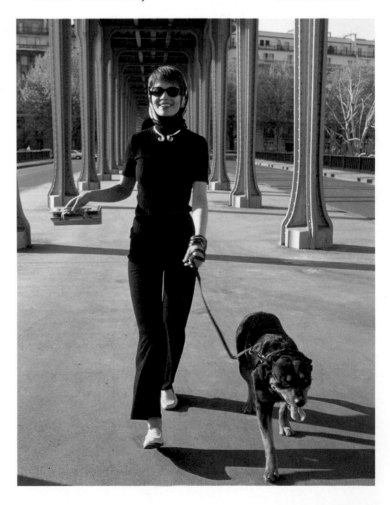

Classic style. You can never have too many pairs of black trousers.

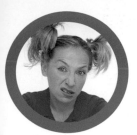

I said in the last chapter that it's easy to go shopping if you are a perfect size 10. But even size 10s have fat days. It is part of the human condition called being female to feel you have suddenly put on half a stone overnight.

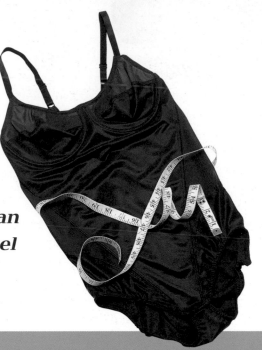

And God created Lycra: beating the bulge

On a rational level you know that you look pretty much the same as you did yesterday and will probably do so tomorrow. However, you're still absolutely certain your tummy looks like you're three months pregnant.

Fortunately, there are ways to make that tummy (and any other fat bits) appear smaller. We're talking fashion magic here! Not just quick fixes, but instant solutions. Yes, you really can slim your thighs, reduce a large bust or make yourself look taller by wearing the right clothes. Conversely, you can add a lot of flab to your figure by wearing the wrong ones, but more of that later. Let's do the good bil first.

When it comes to bums, how low can you go?

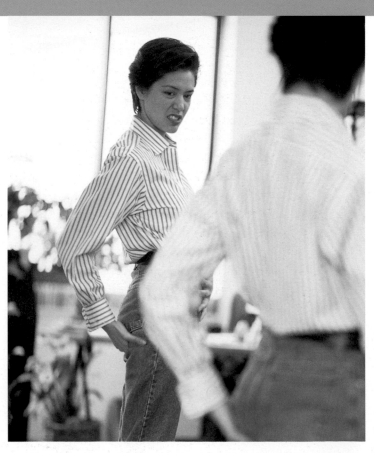

I want to look slimmer now!

Making yourself appear thinner than you really are is all about tricking the eye of your beholder.

RULE 1

Conceal the bits you don't like and high-light the bits you do. That way other people won't even notice your hippo hips, thick ankles or wobbly upper arms. Instead they will be stunned into speechless admiration for your slim neck, tiny waist or well-shaped calves.

In practical terms, this means finding some part of you that is great. If you can't think of anything, then you're being too hard on yourself. Everyone has at least one good feature. Let's say you're a size 24. OK, so you might not like your thighs very much, but chances are you've got a fabulous cleavage. Take pride in it. Get yourself a good bra and wear a top that plunges just a little. If you're too shy, then choose a higher neck but wear a pendant or a scarf over the top. What you're trying to do is focus attention on that great cleavage of yours. Meanwhile, no one's looking at your thighs that you've covered up in loose black trousers.

If, on the other hand, you have a full bust that you hate, but good calves, distract attention away from your top half with a loose, dark coloured tunic and make your calves the main attraction by wearing a mini and sheer tights. A small waist and no bust? Cinch in your waist with an eye-catching belt and stick a Wonderbra on. The list of ways to make the best of your good bits and hide the bad is endless.

If you are a bigger woman, you're probably sick to the back teeth of hearing that phrase, 'But you've got such a lovely face'. I know – I used to be a size 18 and at only five foot tall I looked like a beach ball on legs. People were always patronizing me by saying what nice eyes, lips and ears I had, by which they meant, 'What a shame you can't lose the weight and make the rest of you attractive too'.

However, there is no doubt that some older, bigger women do have the most

beautiful, unlined skin. It really is true what they say about having to choose between your face and your figure after a certain age. It's skinny girls who look raddled as they get older. If you are one of the lucky ones and are wrinkle-free, take some care with your make-up, wear a bright lipstick, try a new hairstyle or a really striking pair of earrings. All of this will encourage people to admire your complexion.

Take a long hard look at yourself in the mirror and work out what your good and bad points are.

RULE 2

Use vertical lines to your advantage. Imagine you are looking at two rooms. One is painted with vertical stripes, the other is plain white. The one with the stripes will appear to have a higher ceiling and be narrower. The white one will seem more spacious, but lower-ceilinged. You can use the same optical effect to shave pounds off yourself.

The most obvious way to use stripes to slim you down is to buy clothes that are striped vertically – a pinstriped trouser suit, for example. Track pants or leggings with stripes down the outside of the leg (you know the brand) are also very flattering. Don't go mad though and get everything striped. You don't want to end up looking like a deckchair.

A subtler approach is to use plain separates to create the vertical lines. A dark coloured jacket worn open over a white tee-shirt, for example, will create the impression of a thick white stripe running down your body – very slimming. A long cardigan over a dress in a contrasting colour works in the same way. Anything V-necked also encourages the viewer's eye to go up and down. Even subtler is using jewellery and accessories. A waist-length string of beads is magically slimming. A long rectangular scarf, worn round the neck then knotted loosely at waist level performs the same trick.

RULE 3

Buy a size larger than you think you need. Nothing makes you look fatter than clothes that cling in all the wrong places. It may give you a high to take a size 12 up to the counter and pay for it, but if you're really a 14, you'll end up looking like a size 16 in a garment that's too small for you. Straining seams, buttons that gape and bits of you bulging out all over the place will make you look fat. End of story.

RULE 4

Buying too large is just as unflattering. Yes, in your fat day depressed state it might be templing to try and hide in a big jumper, but baggy layers make you look larger. The viewer isn't fooled. Shuffle about in acres of extra fabric and onlookers will simply assume that you've got something to hide. Streamlined, but not tight clothing is the best option.

RULE 5

Get yourself some good underwear. These days control garments aren't the iron-clad passion-killers they once were. I'm not saying they're exactly sexy. Let's be honest here. It's a very strange man who finds himself irresistibly drawn to ripping a pair of 40 denier control-top tights off his partner with his teeth. But, thanks to the wonders of Lycra, corsetry is better than it used to be. It's also a heck of a lot more comfortable, whalebone having gone out with the ark.

Control underwear encompasses everything from teeny weeny knickers with a little panel on the front that's supposed to hold you in (does the phrase 'finger in the dyke' mean anything to you?) to full body corsets. Probably the most useful, I think, are control tights because you don't get the

displacement problem (flub exploding out of the bottom) as you sometimes do with control knickers.

If you don't want to go as far as control underwear, you can do a lot for your figure just by wearing the right size of underwear. When trying on a bra, for example, check around the back of your arms to see you're not bulging out there. Another problem area is at the sides of your ribcage. Buy a bra that's too tight there and you create a very ugly roll effect. When it comes to knickers, bigger is definitely better. A smooth line is what you want, so give yourself lots of room. Alternatively, you can go in the opposite direction and buy a G-string. Yes, they're not as comfortable as your big knickers, but they do give you the smoothest possible line under your clothes.

A long jacket is great if you've got big hips.

RULE 6

Wear heels. As a shorty, I'm very pro heels. But, even if you're not five foot nothing, indeed unless you are a six-foot giant, adding even as little as a couple of inches really slims you down. The exceptions are high heels with an ankle strap or ankle boots. Both cut your leg in half making it look fatter. A simple court is much more flattering. If you haven't mastered walking in high heels, get practising.

RULE 7

Stand up straight. It may sound old-fashioned, but good posture really does make you look better. If you slump, you create spare tyres where there weren't any. Remember that old trick about imagining a string coming up through your spine and out the top of your head. Pull the string as tight as you can and feel your back straighten, your neck lengthen and your flab melt away.

RULE 8

Keep your outfit all one colour. I'm not suggesting you wear head-to-toe black, although that probably is the most flattering thing you could do. However, putting together an outfit all in one colour will make you look thinner. The eye of the beholder is encouraged to travel up and down – that vertical line thing again – without interruption.

Still, there are some colours that aren't flattering, even if worn on their own. White is dodgy. White trousers can give you elephant thighs. Red, orange and yellow are also not good. In fact, it's all the warm colours that you have to think twice about. The sort of shades you might chose to paint your living room to make it appear cosy are exactly those that will make you look like an over-stuffed sofa. Cool colours – blues, greens, greys – are more slimming. A darker shade of any colour will also subtract pounds.

Now, just in case you want to know what not to do – or you want to buy something for someone you really really hate and you want her to look dreadful, your partner's ex, for example – here are the things you should avoid like the plague. They're all guaranteed to make you (or her) resemble Ten-Ton Tessie.

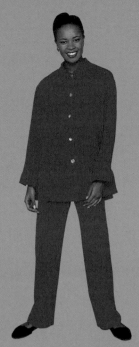

Big can be beautiful. A full, but not stiff, shirt hides a large bust.

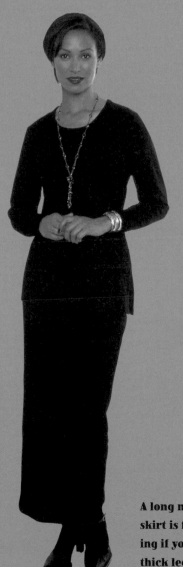

AVOID LIKE THE PLAGUE

horizontal stripes

kaftans

anything sleeveless

anything too tight

ankle boots worn with ankle socks

If you really really hate her, get her a pair of hooped tights. They could make even Naomi Campbell seem hefty legged.

A long narrow skirt is flattering if you've got thick legs.

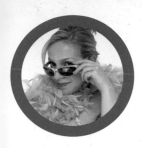

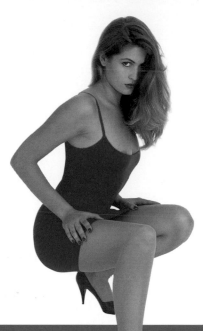

There used to be a question a smug man always asked a woman in the '70s. No, it wasn't, 'Have you burned your bra?', although give him another few pints of Double Diamond and he'd get on to that. No, it was, 'So, do you dress for men or yourself?' If you said you dressed for yourself, he snorted with derision.

Looking for Mr Right (Mr OK in a bad light would do, actually)

If you admitted to sometimes dressing to lure the opposite sex you were branded a traitor to the feminist cause. Mr Smug would make a mental note to bring a bag of his washing round next time he saw you, because you were obviously a closet doormat just aching to look after some chap, any chap really.

The truth is, most women dress for themselves some of the time, for men at other times and attempt a sort of compromise for the rest. If we dressed only for ourselves, we'd all wear leggings and baggy jumpers all the time. We'd never get our roots done and our bosoms would graze our knees as we eschewed bra underwiring in favour of letting it all hang out. Women's lives are complicated. One minute you're a professional dynamo,

another you're a mum, or a handyman, or a chauffeur, etc. Is it any wonder we have complicated wardrobes? We dress according to what we are doing.

There isn't much point in getting togged up to the nines for a trip to the supermarket (unless you fancy acquiring the spotty teenager packing your carriers as a toy boy). That said, when we are going out, we want to dress up a little. Anne Widdicombe aside, most of us would like a sex life. And, sex is like baking a cake. Getting that Victoria sponge to rise does usually require a pinch of something extra. For bicarbonate of soda you can read Wonderbra, sheer stockings, high heels or any of a long list of male turn-ons. Too obvious? Oh, please, you can never be too obvious when it comes to dressing to seduce a man.

26

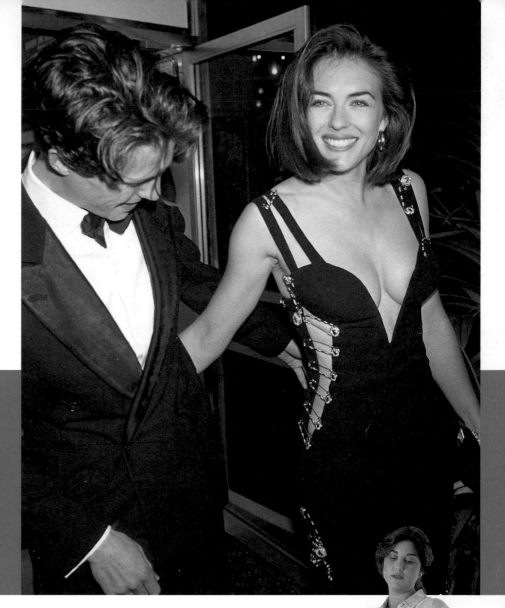

Classy? No. Effective? Absolutely.

The rules of attraction

The male of the species is a pretty basic creature. You could be the president of Mensa with a PhD in applied physics and a Nobel prize for your first novel, but meet a guy at a party and he'll still look down your cleavage. You can rail against this kind of sexism if you like. That is your choice. If you want to ignore every word in this chapter, then flip to the next one. It's just that if you do want to date, there are short cuts, sartorially speaking. If you get to know your male prey, you can hunt so much more effectively.

Colour

The first rule of resultwear, as we shall call it, is to choose the right colour. Here are the colours men hate:

> beige
> green
> black (unless it's a Little Black Dress)
> flesh tones

Yes, there will be blokes who go weak at the knee at the mere glimpse of beige, but they are weird. Get invited home by one of those and you're sure to find he lives with his mother who keeps his dinner warm in the oven while he plays with the points on his Hornby train set in the specially converted garage. Likewise, there will be the odd (very odd) chap who likes flesh tones. He's the one hanging round phone boxes writing down numbers.

The reason most men dislike beige is that it is a mummy colour. It is comfy, cosy, unexciting, asexual – the sort of thing they might imagine their mum wearing. The same goes for flesh tones. As a small child, they are sure to have seen some of their mother or grandmother's smalls hanging on a washing line. And, what colour are old-fashioned girdles? Why, flesh, of course. Unless you have firm plans to open a bed and breakfast hotel for grown men who enjoy wearing nappies, avoid flesh-coloured clothing.

'Where on earth can he be? Was it something I did?' The dire consequences of wearing beige.

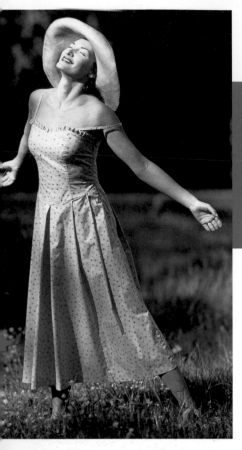

Like a virgin.
Spriggy prints
for the would-
be wife.

The aversion to green is pure superstition. Just as many women won't wear it, so many men associate it with bad luck too. As for black, one of the commonest male refrains of the last 10 years has to be, 'Haven't you got anything in your wardrobe besides black?' Blokes don't understand that you want your thighs to look less hefty, they simply think black is dreary. The exception to this rule is evening wear, when black suddenly becomes sultry, mysterious and elegant, or maybe they've just had a few extra vodkas.

Now you know what colours NOT to wear if you want to get yourself a date. Here are the surefire winners:

**red
white
pastels
floral prints**

Red is the colour of fire, passion and sex. In the male brain, a woman who sports scarlet is automatically a tigress just waiting to undo his flies with her teeth. She's hot stuff! Red should, therefore, be handled with caution. You need the confidence to pull it off. Practise a dismissive curl of the lip perhaps. Certainly, prepare yourself for the distinct possibility that, if you do pull, he'll expect you to walk up and down his chest in high heels. If you are a shrinking

violet, it might be wise to work up to a full-on postbox hue. Start off with a pink or a burgundy.

White carries the opposite, but no-less-potent, message. White is the colour of innocence and virginity. Yes, these days a chap has to be pretty optimistic to think that a woman, even if she is wearing white, might actually be an innocent virgin. Still,

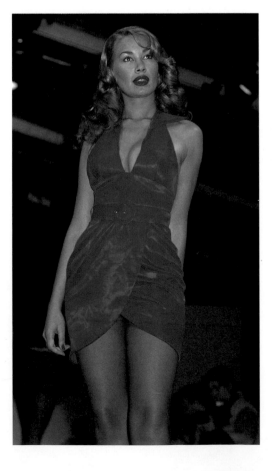

Short and not too sweet. He'll definitely buy you a drink, but you might not be invited home to meet his mum.

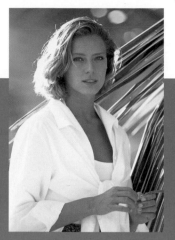

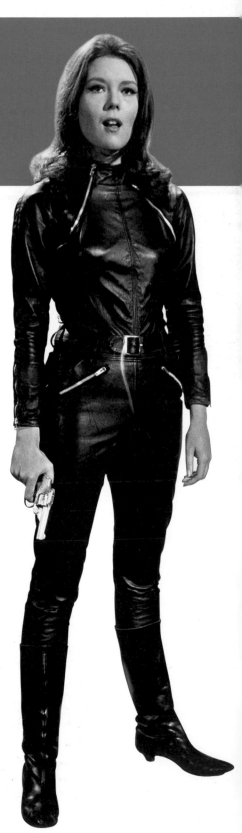

he can dream, can't he? White works particularly well if you are looking for a more traditional, chivalrous kind of chap.

To a lesser extent, the same goes for pastel colours and floral prints. Again, we're talking you as fragile flower, him as strong protector. If you're not that fragile a flower, then pastels and florals might be a better bet than pure white. You're stretching credibility less. A word of warning, though. If you're going to tog yourself up as a snowy-hued virgin or a spriggy lily of the valley, it's a good idea to remember your manners. Swearing like a navvy or chain smoking like Bradford during the Industrial Revolution blow the effect.

Touchability

I'm going to stick up for men here. It is said that men are primarily a visual gender. Certainly, they respond to visual cues, but to describe them as only visual is crude and unfair. Many guys are also highly tactile. Perhaps it's because they are denied the chance to wear nice soft fabrics themselves that many love the feeling of feminine fabrics. Wearing slithery satin, flimsy silk, or fluffy velvet or velour can be a real turn-on. All encourage a man to want to touch you, with your permission of course.

Leather and PVC are also highly effective, if a bit explosive. No, you won't necessarily attract a man who spends his lunch hours being locked in a box by someone who calls herself Madame Sin. Even normal(ish) guys like the idea of a woman in leather. Why else was *The Avengers* so popular? If you want to lure a leather fancier rather than the aficionado, make it a leather mini rather than a leather bra.

The push-pull principle

It seems a tad obvious (but then what did I say about men and being obvious?) but the male of the species is attracted to the female because she is different from him. Girls have bosoms and waists and hips. We might wish we had a bit less of any of these, but most men are quite happy with us as we are. Given the choice between the Mae West/Marilyn Monroe type and Twiglet woman, most guys would choose the former.

So, don't hide your light under a bushel. Be proud of what you have and pull it in and push it up. Piling on baggy sweatshirts and wearing dungarees or voluminous dresses is easy and comfortable. However, they will kill your sex appeal. So get that Wonderbra on and climb into those support tights. If your body's up to it, try a clingy Lycra skirt and top. If not, go for tailored garments that follow the line of your body.

How to make yourself into a man magnet

Now you know a few basic rules, it's time to talk specifics. Which outfits will guarantee you get a date? In reverse order, here are my top 10 resultwear combos:

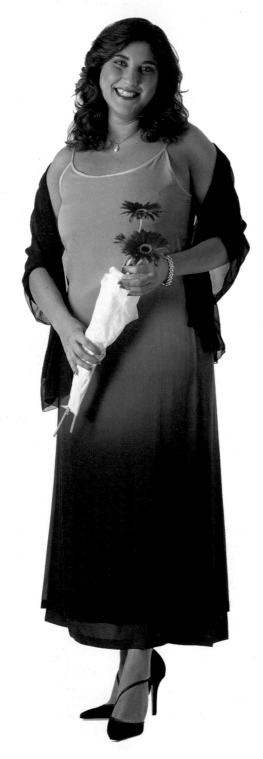

When floaty equals flirty. The essential summer dress.

10

Long, floaty summer dress with shoe-string straps

The floatiness of the dress and the length of the skirt give this outfit a demure feel: it's a bit vicar's daughter. What could be dull is made sexy, however, by the shoe-string straps. They offer the tantalizing possibility that they might slip and your whole dress fall off. Unlikely, perhaps, but in the fevered male brain such scenarios are always just a gust of wind away.

9

Long slit or wrap-over skirt with crisp white shirt

The crisp white cotton of the shirt and the length of the skirt produce a slightly schoolmarm look. It's the Virginia Bottomley effect. To the right guy, one who wants to be bossed about a bit, this look is manna (or should that be mama) from heaven. The slit in the skirt offers little glimpses of the delights that lurk beneath.

8

Long evening dress with plunge back

Plunge backs are more unusual than plunge fronts. Because your bosoms stay safely covered, a backless frock is regarded as classier, particularly if it is long. What makes it sexy, however, is the amount of flesh on display – a lot – and the fact that while you can get a strapless bra under a scoop-front dress, a backless dress is proof you're not wearing one. Ooh, missus.

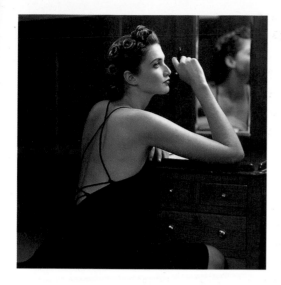

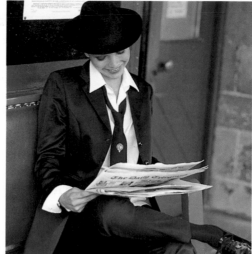

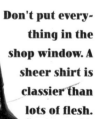

7

Sheer blouse with buttons up the front, above the knee skirt and high heels

This is pretty standard secretary wear – a notebook and glasses are optional acces-sories – and so taps into the whole 'Oh, Miss Jones, you're beautiful' male fantasy. The fact that the blouse is sheer and so offers a hint of the underwear beneath gives it an extra element of sex appeal.

6

Long knitted dress with zip-up front

Anything that zips up is a real winner. A guy can work out immediately how he might get it off, which lessens the performance pres-sure should he succeed in getting you into that situation. The knitted (you could try jersey) dress clings to your curves.

5

Man's suit and tie

Remember the ad for men's shirts that fea-tured a shot of a woman in a shirt? It read: 'It looks even better on a man.' Actually, most chaps would disagree. Masculine clothes point up a woman's femininity. One word of caution, though. If you are going to wear a tie, keep it at half-mast, otherwise he'll think you are a lesbian.

4

Leather jeans and tee-shirt

Not all men like women to be too dressed up. The tee-shirt suggests you're laid back. The rock-chick leather jeans suggest that you could, however, be stirred into action if necessary.

3

Jeans and cropped top

This is a less frightening version of the leather jeans and tee-shirt. The image is less rock chick than sporty girl next door. He likes it because you are flashing a little flesh and he can see what he's getting. The upside for you is that it's com-fortable. The downside is that you have to do sit-ups.

2

Short skirt with anything

Men suffer from selective blindness. Wear a mini and they won't notice whether you've got good cheekbones, fine wrists or a nice smile. All they see is legs. And they won't even notice if your pins are not that good either, within reason.

1

Short red dress

Chris de Burgh wrote a song about it. 'Nuff said.

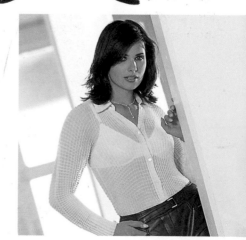

Rock chick chic (if you've got the legs that is).

Don't put every-thing in the shop window. A sheer shirt is classier than lots of flesh.

SO YOU WANT TO BE IN ON A SATURDAY NIGHT?

Just in case you want to know how to repel all male admirers, here's my top 10 male turn-offs.

10 DUNGAREES – HE THINKS YOU'RE A LESBIAN **9** TWEED SUIT – HE THINKS YOU'RE HIS MOTHER **8** KAFTAN – HE THINKS YOU'RE DEMIS ROUSSOS **7** KNEE-LENGTH SKIRT AND POP SOCKS – TOTALLY UNSEXY **6** CULOTTES – THE ONLY SHORTS HE LIKES ARE HOT PANTS **5** TWINSET – TOO MUMSY AGAIN **4** TRACKSUIT – SLOVENLY **3** OPAQUE TIGHTS – HE REGARDS THEM AS ONLY A SHADE OFF SURGICAL STOCKINGS **2** LEGGINGS – YOU WANT HIM TO THINK YOU'RE NOT MAKING AN EFFORT? **1** BAGGY JUMPER – HE THINKS YOU MUST BE REALLY FAT UNDERNEATH

Now you are fully apprised of everything you need to know to hook the man of your dreams – well almost. There are complications. The clothes a man likes to see you in vary according to what stage of the relationship you have reached. You need to fine tune your wardrobe accordingly.

Whetting his appetite

This is the eyes meeting across a crowded room stage. It's where you're getting dressed for a party or a club. You are going out to get a date, so you need to be at your sexiest. We're talking little red dress, Little Black Dress, high heels and plunging top.

OK, he called

If and when you have a first date, you need to think carefully about what to wear. It is tempting just to choose the thing in your wardrobe that makes you look thinnest. This isn't necessarily the best option. You need to consider where you are going for your date – a movie date means a different outfit from a posh candlelight dinner date – and remember what you were wearing when you first met him.

If he was attracted to you when you were wearing a scarlet leather catsuit, it's probably best not to put on a tracksuit for date one. He'll think you are schizophrenic. What you want to aim for is a subtler version of the look that initially attracted him. The setting is more intimate and, frankly, he doesn't want to see your cleavage over dinner.

You've already established that you are drop dead gorgeous, now you want him to get to know you better. Jeans and a simple top are fantastic if it's an early evening movie date – you look as if you're not trying too hard. For anything posher, the Little Black Dress (LBD) is a great standby – smart but not showy. If you're going out straight from work, you could try replacing your normal office shirt with a sheer tee-shirt. That said, I did once try this ruse. My date waited till the end of the evening then said: 'Why are you wearing a net curtain?'

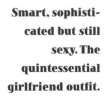

Smart, sophisticated but still sexy. The quintessential girlfriend outfit.

Now you're his girlfriend

When you're first dating, he invariably wants you to look sexy. It impresses his friends for one thing. When you become his official girlfriend, however, everything changes. All of a sudden he wants you to don a yashmak. This is incredibly irritating, but entirely understandable. Men are insecure. He thinks that unless you are wearing a tent over your head, you might run off with somebody else, and he doesn't want you to do that. Indeed, if you do have a row over a short skirt, take heart. The uglier and more asexual he wants you to look, the more committed to you he is.

You don't have to go down the yashmak route; just throttle back a little on the minis and cleavage. Go for smart and sophisticated, not slutty.

My wife and I

If and when you become his wife, he will want you to be even more demure. The preferred look is sort of BA stewardess chic – polished and professional-looking, sexy but unavailable. You know when you have got to this state when he starts pointing at low-heeled court shoes and saying how nice he thinks they'd look on you.

Remember, in all this you have a choice. You can wear whatever you like. That is your right. It's just that if you understand the way your man thinks, not only are you likely to have fewer rows about clothes, he might actually buy you a few. Remember knowledge is power!

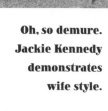

Oh, so demure. Jackie Kennedy demonstrates wife style.

Sharon Stone. Fine as fantasy, but you try going out without knickers on and he'll get his in a right old twist.

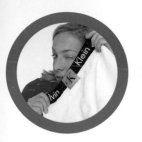

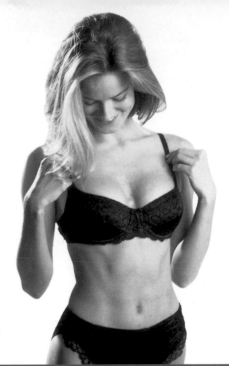

If you get your resultwear right, there will come a point when you will have to appear naked in fron of someone else – him. This is a traumatic point in any relationsh

Sex and the single spare tyre

The one reason more than any other that-women stay in bad relationships is that they just can't bear the thought of someone new seeing their cellulite. The current squeeze may be a total pig, but at least he doesn't laugh when you take your clothes off. Still, there is a way to make the garment removal less hideous and that's to get your underwear right.

I can't be that big!

Women are often told off for not buy-ing the right size of underwear. Various figures are bandied about. Up to 50 % of us are supposed to be wear-ing the wrong size. The inference is that the British woman walks around lingerie departments in a daze, picking up anything she sees without checking the size. Then, when she gets it home and puts it on, she is too dim to notice it doesn't fit.

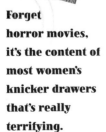

Forget horror movies, it's the content of most women's knicker drawers that's really terrifying.

It may be comfy, but is it sexy?

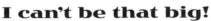

The truth is, if a lot of us are wearing underwear that is too big or too small, it's because we are forced into it by an industry that simply doesn't cater for those at the top and bottom end of the size range. Yes, they say they do, but you try finding a pretty 34 E-cup bra! 'Needle' and 'haystack' are words that come to mind. If you don't wear a 34B bra and standard-size knickers, then it's difficult to buy nice lingerie. When you get past a D-cup, shoulder straps widen and lace becomes cheap-looking. Marks and Spencer do the occa-sional style in a size bigger than a D. Their minimizer bras are also good. Otherwise, if you're an awkward size, try department stores. The Triumph and Fantasie labels do a pretty extensive range of sizes. If you do visit a department store and can't see anything in your size, ask an assistant to help. They might be able to order what you need. And don't forget

34

about mail order. OK, some of the stuff would make Hyacinth Bucket's smalls look like the height of fashion – I had no idea that the corselette still existed – but at least you can try things on in the privacy of your own bedroom and send them back if they don't fit.

As a last resort there is always the option of paying a fortune and visiting a posh corsetière, where you will be properly fitted. When I was a size 18, an E-cup and at the end of my tether I went to one of these places. Lots of posh people were supposed to buy their knickers from this shop, so it must be good I thought.

I went into the cubicle and took my top off and a very stern woman came in and inspected me. It reminded me of the nit inspections we used to have at school. I expected to hear the clink of a metal comb against the side of a metal kidney bowl of disinfectant at any moment. 'Well,' my fitter snorted, 'you can't wear your bosoms as high as that, madam.' A bit of a row ensued, during which I told her that I could wear my bosoms as eye-patches if I chose. Finally I calmed down, tried on a selection of flesh-coloured garments with straps the width of the M4 and ended up buying the least offensive one. It cost £27 and was completely hideous and totally unsexy. I never wore it.

So, be fitted by all means (you can get this done in any good department store, and even at M&S), but don't expect it to solve your problems. It could be the start of a long and thankless search.

Hoisting them up

I have a girlfriend whose mother told her to wear a bra 24 hours a day. She has followed her mother's advice for the whole of her adult life, only removing her bra in the

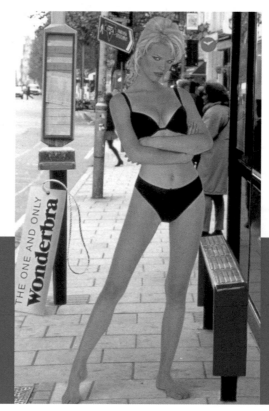

OK, you're proud of your cleavage, but put some clothes on, love.

bath or, on special occasions, in bed. Still, at 35 she has the most fabulously uplifted cleavage. The rest of us, who were not taught the benefits of 24-hour bra wearing, need a bit more help and this is where underwiring comes in.

The person who invented underwiring should be canonized. This patron saint of the perky frontage has done us all the most immense favour. That said, there are two downsides to the underwired bra:

1   The wires can work loose. Then they either stab you under the arms – there is no pain like it – or knacker your washing machine.

2   When you take your bra off, your breasts are apt to tumble downwards at an alarming rate. At this point one ex-boyfriend of mine used to shout 'timber' like a lumberjack.

Hoisting them up even further

There is a way to boost the effects of an underwired bra. It's not exactly comfortable but if you want to wear your bosoms as a necklace, give it a go.

What you do is deliberately buy the wrong size bra. You choose one that is a size larger round the ribs but smaller in the cup than you would normally buy. When you put your new bra on, you then tighten the shoulder straps as far as they will go. As a result, the whole bra will sit higher on your rib cage (it can because you've bought it a size larger round the chest) and the little cups will force your bosoms up and out.

As I said, it's not comfortable and no doubt I'll get appalled letters from bra-fitters across the land. But the girl who taught me this trick is never short of a boyfriend, so who cares?

When underwiring just isn't enough

So, you've got your underwired bra and it still isn't giving you the oomph you want. Time to get serious about pumping up that cleavage. First option is a padded push-up bra. The Wonderbra and Ultrabra are both excellent, although you have to be careful you don't lose the pads. They can work themselves free of their little pouches and you can leave a trail of them behind you if you're not careful.

Another idea are those little semicircles of sticky cardboard that you can buy from department stores. You stick one semicircle under each breast and they sort of prop them up. Do they work? Yes, but your date gets a heck

of a shock if you forget to nip to the bathroom to remove them before retiring to the sofa for a nightcap.

More terrifying still are silicon implants. I don't mean surgery here, although that is pretty scary. Rather, those jelly-like cushions that you slip inside your bra. Again, they're available from department stores. They give a very natural look – until you remove your clothing. Then they look about as natural as a bag of frozen peas shoved down your bra. Actually, they can feel quite cold next to your skin and, as they aren't part of you and have no blood running through them, can stay feeling cold no matter how hot under the collar you get.

The Sellotape trick

This is much used by models on photo sessions and is great if you're wearing a dress under which you can't put a bra. It's not very ladylike though.

First, grab hold of your bosoms and push them up and together. Hold them in position with one hand. With the other hand, take a roll of Sellotape and, beginning under one armpit, run the tape across

Fabulous frontage. A good fit is essential.

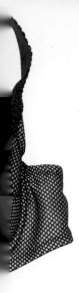

When in doubt, push them up. The benefits of underwiring.

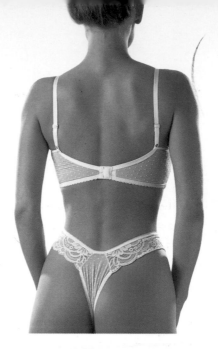

How to avoid VPL. The cheesewire effect of a G-string.

and under your breasts to the other armpit. Rip off the end of the tape. Repeat this several times, going backwards and forwards until you don't need to hold your bosoms any more. They stay up on their own. Go as high up your breasts and as far into your armpits as you can – it will be more secure – but not so far that the tape will show under your frock.

It takes a few times to master the Sellotape trick. Getting a girl-friend to help you is a good idea, if the pair of you can stop laughing long enough to do it, that is. Also, if you have sensitive skin, be warned. You might be allergic to the glue in the tape. (When I did this once, I came out in

nasty pink stripes like a diseased zebra.) If you are allergic, get hold of some toupée tape instead. The glue is less virulent.

Lingerie and lurve

Most girls have two sets of lingerie. The first is the comfy stuff. If you're single, you wear this when you're on your own. If you're attached, you wear it all the time, except when he really really begs you to wear stockings and suspenders.

It is amazing how Pavlovian (I mean the dogs not the meringue dessert here) blokes are about stockings. I have never met a guy who didn't go doolally over them. You can be po-faced about it if you like. There is no law that says you have to truss yourself up like a chicken just because that's what he finds attractive, but consider this: stockings and suspenders are great camouflage. If you are worried about your flabby thighs and you put on stockings and suspenders, he'll be so riveted by them, he won't notice anything else.

The things we do for love. Trussed up like a chicken for a special night.

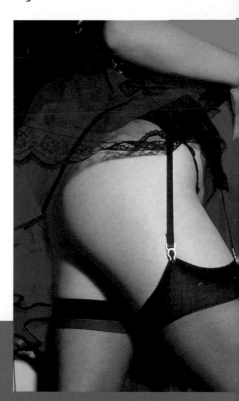

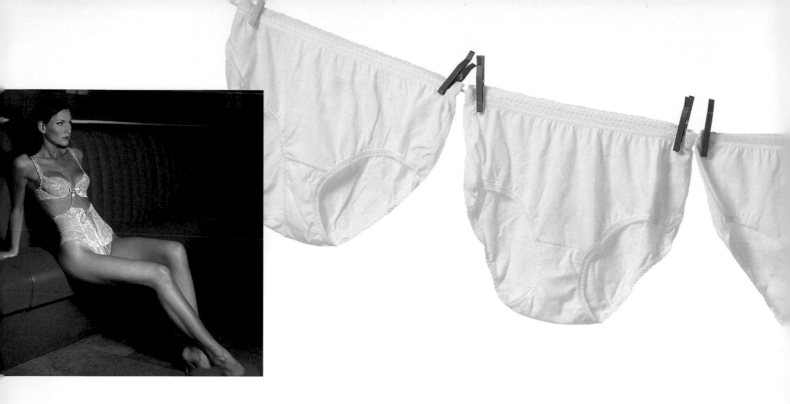

Yes, big knickers can be glamorous.

If you want to go the whole hog and drive him berserk between the sheets, here is the complete list of things men find sexy, lingerie-wise:

> suspenders
> hold-up stockings
> high heels (yes, in bed)
> G-strings
> red satin
> black PVC
> white lace

We've talked about suspenders already. If you really hate them, you could give hold-up stockings a go. I once met a model who complained that she couldn't wear hold-ups because 'they always slip down on me'. I hated her immediately. Imagine having thighs so waif-like that hold-ups fall down! The problem with hold-ups is quite the opposite for most of us. Hold-ups have the unfortunate habit of squeezing the thighs so tightly that flesh bulges out over the top. This can make your legs look like pasty strings of sausages. As for wearing high heels in bed – at only five foot tall, I need all the help I can get.

Got a bottom you want to hide? Try loose French knickers.

G-strings are a contentious subject. The first time you put one on it will be very very uncomfortable. However, not only do they eliminate the Visible Panty Line (VPL), they are also sexy and – this is a very big AND – they can make your bottom look smaller. It's that vertical line thing again. On colour, you should observe the same rules as resultwear – red, black and white. The PVC option is for the brave.

Just in case you never want to date again, here is the definitive list of man-repelling underwear:

> anything in a flesh tone
> big knickers
> opaque tights

I was talking to a woman who confessed that when she puts on her flesh-coloured tee-shirt bra her husband has to close his eyes. He hates the sight of her in that bra that much. If you want to turn him off, wear it by all means.

Another massive no-no is big knickers. Yes, we love them. They hold everything in and they're really comfy. Blokes loathe them for the same reasons. They cover everything up and are

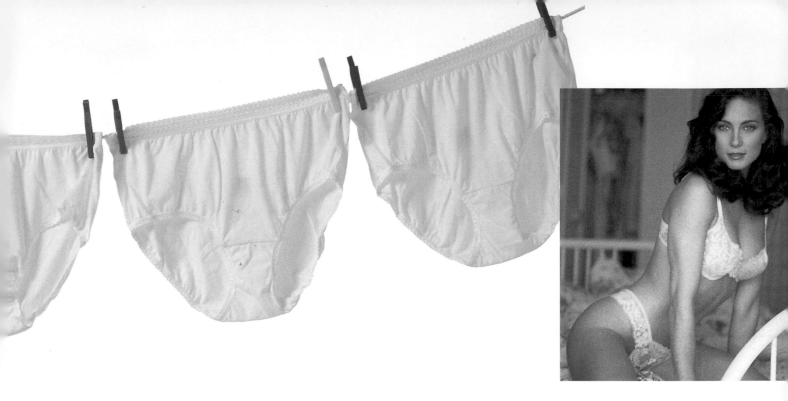

murder to get off. Plus, they remind them of their mum's or their granny's knickers. French knickers, the satin baggy kind, are almost as bad. The rule for sexy knickers really is less is more.

Tights are a turn-off in general, but opaque tights are especially contraceptive. Again, we love them because they cover everything. Men just don't get it. 'Like a sack of spuds' is how one male acquaintance described a woman's bottom in opaque tights. Guys associate them with support stockings and Zimmer frames and, well, just don't wear them on a date.

The five-date rule

There is a way to use unsexy lingerie to your advantage. As all clever girls know, you should never sleep with a man on the first date. Date five is the correct one at which to get to know him better. This is great in theory, but this is the '90s. How does a red-blooded girl stop herself succumbing on date three or four? She wears unsexy underwear that's how.

When you feel yourself wavering, you put on your most unsexy underwear – the greying bra, the knickers that went pink in the wash, the tights that have a knot in the waistband since the elastic went. As an extra safety net, you do not shave your legs or under your arms. Then, if your virtue weakens, your vanity will save you because you will be too embarrassed to take off your clothes in case he sees your awful grungy underwear. (Now, why did they never teach me that in my school sex education lessons. It would have been far more useful than the reproduction system of the tape worm.)

Worried about your tummy? Try a teddy.

You've spent a fortune on sexy lingerie and you're still worried about your cellulite

You can kit yourself out in La Perla outfits for every day of the week, but at some point they're going to have to come off, right? Wrong. The best thing about choosing really fabulous lingerie is that you can keep it on in bed. You get to keep all the bits you hate covered up and he thinks you're incredibly adventurous.

Need a bit of uplift? Keep your bra on.

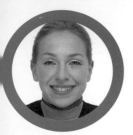

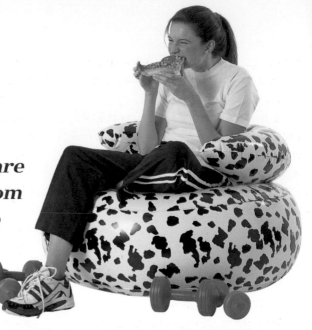

Do you like mustard? Colman's are supposed to have got rich not from the mustard we eat, but from the amount everybody leaves on the side of their plate. Gyms operate on the same principle.

Gym fascism
(do I have to wear a leotard ?)

It's not the people actually puffing on the treadmill who make gym owners money, it's everybody else who went once, paid their subscriptions and then couldn't bear ever to go again. The same goes for the makers of fitness books, cassettes and videos. They're making a mint out of us NOT using their stuff.

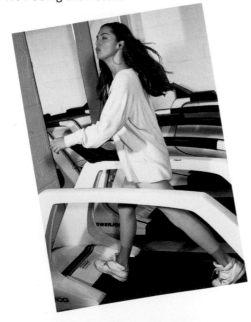

If you don't know what to wear to the gym, you can't go wrong with a big tee-shirt.

So why do we do this – waste our money? Here are my top five reasons not to go to the gym:

1   Everybody is going to be thin and gorgeous and you're going to feel like a heffalump.
2   You won't know how to use any of the equipment and you'll make a total fool of yourself.
3   You'll have to put on a leotard.
4   You'll have to have a 'fitness assessment' and that means being weighed in public.
5   You'd rather sit on the sofa and eat pizza.

There is no doubt that every gym has its quota of thin and gorgeous women. They're the ones who strut about in fluorescent leo-tards with a G-string back and contrasting cycle shorts. But ask yourself how come they've got all that free time to strut about? Could it be that they don't have a job, a boyfriend, any kids, a life?

Actually, I was in a gym once in Paris and it was full of those kind of women. One was on the Stairmaster and she was wearing a complete outfit – real clothes, not exercise gear – and shoes with bows on. With bows on! She spent her entire time looking at herself in the mirror. I'd like to say she fell off the Stairmaster or some other hideous accident befell her. Sadly it didn't. I just didn't go back to that gym again. (Yeah, I do it too.)

Most gyms, though, are filled with women just like you – women who are battling with a hippopotamus bottom or elephant thighs. And no, they're not all staring at you. Frankly, exercising is hellish enough without extending the amount of time you have to do it by wasting precious minutes staring at other people.

Reassuringly, every gym also has its enormously fat quota too. There is always someone bigger than you. I was once in a gym in London – the story of me and my thighs is an ongoing one – and the token very large woman walked up to me. This was a bit rude because I had just come out of the shower and was stark naked. She looked me up and down slowly and said: 'You look slimmer on the TV.' Then she walked off. No, I didn't go back to that gym again either.

The likelihood that you will be insulted when in the nude is pretty low. What is more worrying for most of us is not knowing how to use the battery of equipment in a gym. The good news is that you don't have to know. You don't have to use it if you don't want to. If you are a techno whizz, the treadmill that talks to you and the bike with space-age dials might be your bag. But it's not fancy machines that get you fit, it's you. You can stick to the skipping rope and do some press-ups and get just as fit.

If you think using the machines will work for you, ask an assistant for help. That's what they're there for, remember. It's in their interests to explain things clearly to you, otherwise you might sue the gym if you slip a disc. Before you ever get on to any machine, you should get a proper demonstration. This means you needn't ever be in the position of not knowing what to do and making a total fool of yourself.

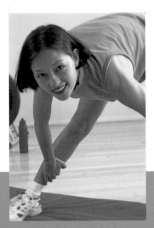

Exercise doesn't have to be high tech. The oldest exercises are the best.

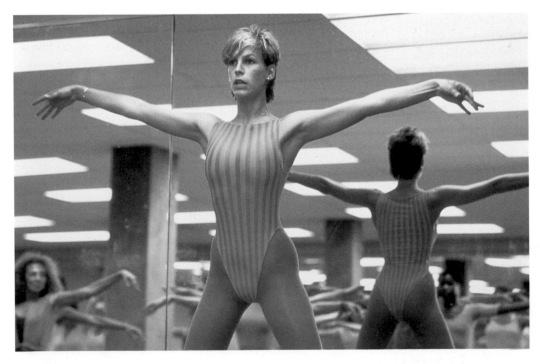

Jamie Lee Curtis in 'Perfect' shape. Don't you just hate her?

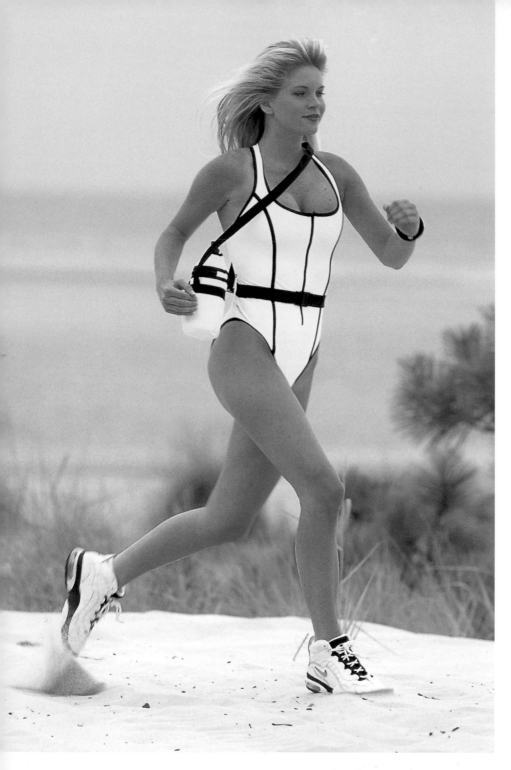

Beach babe, aka the woman every other girl would love to throttle.

scales and gives you a lecture on healthy eating. But the thing to remember here is that, again, they're covering their backs. Just in case you turn round and have a heart attack, they can tell your grieving family that it wasn't their fault as you didn't tell them you had a dicky heart at your fitness assessment.

It is precisely the point at which you are standing on those scales that you start fantasizing about sitting on the sofa and eating pizza. And, certainly, that is a lifestyle option. The problem is if you did that all the time, then you might end up like one of those American women who has to be lifted out of bed by a crane and taken to hospital to have her jaws wired together. The crane bit isn't so bad. It's the fact she's always wearing a really horrible tracksuit that's embarrassing.

Reasons to go to the gym

1   You might lose some weight.
2   Er, that's it actually.

There is only one reason to go to the gym and that's to shift a spare tyre. Anyone who starts burbling on about wanting to have a healthier lifestyle is lying. They're just panicking about a wobbly bottom or chunky midriff.

You don't have to go to a gym to lose weight. I mean, I'd still rather shave my eyebrows than go on a Stairmaster. You could 'incorporate exercise into your lifestyle'. Health gurus are always suggesting that. 'At work,' they say, 'take the stairs instead of the lift.' Or they suggest, 'On the way home, get off the bus a few stops early.' Fine in theory, not so great in practice.

What if the reason you need to go up a couple of floors in the office lift is that you've got a document you need to get to

The wearing a leotard bit is not essential. But more of that later. Let's deal with the psychological issues first. This brings us to the so-called 'fitness assessment'. This has to be the cruellest blow to potential gym-goers. You get up the courage to walk through the door of your local fitness establishment and the first thing they do is hand you over to a teenager on work experience who makes you stand on a pair of your boss in a hurry. I can't see many bosses being happy to hang about while you 'incorporate exercise into your lifestyle'. Likewise, getting off the bus before you need to is a bit tricky if you're carrying a week's shopping or have a gaggle of small children and a pushchair with you. If you have the time to 'incorporate exercise into your lifestyle', you've probably got time to go to a proper gym.

GYM FASHION NO-NOS

BRIGHTLY PATTERNED LEOTARDS • G-STRING-BACKED LEOTARDS • CYCLE SHORTS • FLESH-COLOURED LEGGINGS • CROPPED TOPS AND TIE-WAIST TRACK PANTS • SHELLSUITS • TRACKSUITS

Leotard hell

It is one of life's great ironies that a woman only ever puts on a leotard when she knows she has to lose weight. And yet a leotard only ever looks good on you when you don't have a pound to lose. The thought of climbing into one of these horrible garments has to be the single biggest reason why women don't go to the gym. We try on a leotard in the privacy of our own homes and are so disgusted with the way we look in it that we can't bring ourselves to inflict this vision on anyone else.

Exercise wear, by its very nature, is un-flattering. It is either very tight – little Lycra tops and cycle shorts – and so clings to every roll of fat, or it is very baggy – track-suits – and makes you look like a barrage balloon. Still, there are ways to make it look a whole lot better. Let's start with what you should avoid.

Anything patterned adds inches. Make it bright and patterned and not only will you look bigger, but you'll be drawing attention to the fact. You might as well hang a flashing sign round your neck that says: 'I like ice-cream and I've got the tummy to prove it.' A G-string-backed leotard and cycle shorts are another brutal combination. If you look like Elle McPherson, give it a go. If you don't, steer clear. There is nowhere for any excess flesh to hide.

The two most unflattering bottom halves you could go for are flesh-coloured leggings – very fattening – and tie-waisted track pants. You see the latter worn with a cropped top a lot. On the perfectly toned, this outfit looks great. But tie-waists are bulky and unless you have the body of Jamie Lee Curtis you will look like a sack of potatoes. You can go in the opposite direction and opt for things that are really baggy all over. However, this can be just as unflattering. Shellsuits and tracksuits scream 'I hate my body!' They add inches all over, taking away any shape you have.

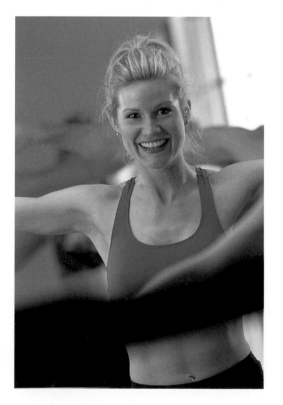

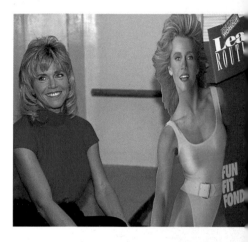

Oh dear, Jane. Nice pectorals, shame about the eye make-up.

She's got a toned midriff, but she doesn't have to look so smug about it.

FLATTERING EXERCISE WEAR

LEOTARDS AND LEGGINGS THAT MATCH ● BIG TEE-SHIRTS AND LEGGINGS ● TRACK PANTS WITH UNCUFFED HEMS ● TRACK PANTS WITH STRIPES DOWN THE SIDE

If you can't be bothered to hold your tummy in, bung a baggy top over it.

OK, there is no such thing as truly flattering exercise wear, but you can be a bit kinder to your body if you pick carefully. First off, choose an outfit all in one colour. A leotard and leggings that match are much more flattering than mismatching pieces. Obviously, a dark colour also helps. If you can't bear to wear a leotard, you could go for a big tee-shirt. But remember, you're adding a lot of bulk with all that fabric. You could be making yourself appear plumper than you are.

The key is to isolate which bits of you need covering and which are OK. Go tight with Lycra where you can and baggy everywhere else. If you have good legs but a big torso, try a baggy tee-shirt and leggings. If it's your hips and legs that are the problem, go tight on the top half and baggy around the bottom.

Track pants are ideal for hiding heavy legs. Choose ones with as little gathering round the waist as possible and no cuffs at the ankle. Straight-legged jogging bottoms are much more slimming than loose, cuffed ones. If you can find a pair with stripes running down the side, even better. Team these with a tighter top half – go for a top with cap sleeves if you're worried about your arms – or a top with a scoop neck.

When buying exercise wear, it's tempting just to take it off the rack and pay for it. But unless you're buying just a loose tee-shirt, you must try it on. And make sure you

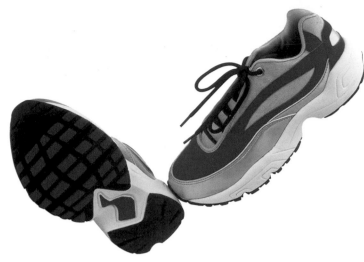

try it on while wearing an exercise bra. Aerobics classes are full of girls who didn't do this. Their tops look OK from the front, but from the back they scoop down, revealing every greying, unsexy strap of their exercise bra.

On the subject of exercise bras, they are essential. There is no point working like a Trojan to get a gorgeous bum, only for your bosoms to sink south in the process. Of the two types available, bra strap-style and racer back, the former will give you much better support. If you are larger busted, consider wearing more than one. You'll feel less embarrassed if you're not wobbling about as you exercise.

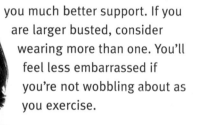

Ugly, but essential: a good sports bra.

Au naturel? You must be joking

However hard you try to find nice fitness clothing, chances are you're still going to feel you're not really looking your best at the gym – and that's before 20 minutes of Callanetics. As with all crisis situations, one way to make yourself feel better is to put on make-up. No, I'm not suggesting a full Joan Collins job. Start a step aerobics class in that and by the end of it you'll look like Alice Cooper. However, there is no reason why you can't wear a bit of make-up.

Foundation should be avoided. As you sweat it sort of slides down and you'll be left with a beige rim around your tee-shirt. Lipstick looks OK. However, if you are doing frantic movements there is always the possibility you will brush your mouth with one hand. Have you seen Jack Nicholson as The Joker in *Batman*? Better do without the lippy. You won't need blusher either, as you should be working up a bit of colour anyway. Still, you can apply waterproof mascara and a little lip gloss. Not much, but enough to lift your spirits.

One last tip on the fitness fashion front: if you want to make your legs looks slimmer – and who doesn't? – buy a pair of clompy trainers. The bigger your shoes, the more pipe-cleaneresque your legs will look. Don't go mad though. Trying to run four miles in Spice Girl platform trainers is not only difficult, it's downright dangerous.

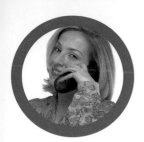

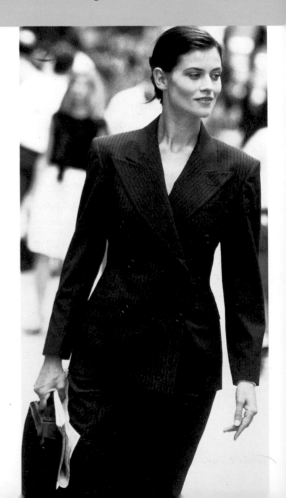

It is often said that people make up their mind about you within 30 seconds of meeting you. If they do, on what basis are they making their judgement? On the way you look, of course. Now, this isn't nice and it certainly isn't fair.

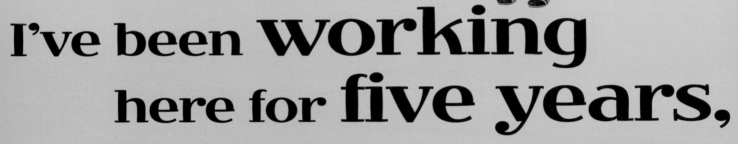

I've been working here for five years,

so how come I'm still the one who has to buy the Hobnobs?

The person being dismissed as a nerd could be the brightest, funniest man on earth. It's just that he really should curb his taste in tank tops. As for the woman with the purple mascara, maybe she's kind to animals and old people. Shame about the make-up, though.

On a social level, such snap judgements are annoying. In a professional situation, however, they can be devastating. A good or bad first impression can make the difference between being hired or not, getting a promotion or being passed over, securing a pay rise or having to take a pay cut. Of course, the quality of your work and the way you relate to others are important. But only a fool would underestimate the part appearance plays in professional advancement. How many skinheads do you see at the CBI annual conference?

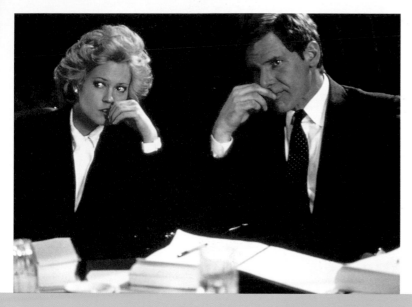

**Working Girl:
Melanie Griffiths
borrows the boss's
clothes to get to
the top.**

Getting started

It's a horrible American phrase, but you really can 'dress for success' and the first step is to decide what message you want to get across. If you work for a city bank, then being a bit flash is par for the course. You need to convey confidence, almost cockiness. This translates as designer labels, bright colours and jokey accessories. Try the same look behind the desk of the local DSS, where trustworthiness and at least a hint of a caring attitude are expected, and you probably wouldn't make it through your first day.

But don't get carried away and overdo the executive dressing bit. Your work clothes also need to be practical. If you are driving a bus or running a playgroup, there isn't much point in wearing high heels and a power suit. Think about how much time you will spend standing up. Is a lot of hard physical work involved in your job? Will you be going out and meeting clients? Choose clothes that, at the very least, do not hinder you doing a good job. For example, if you are a rep who does a lot of driving and therefore would rather not wear heels, wear flats by all means. Before you go into meetings, simply swap these for a pair of smart courts you keep in the glove compartment.

Looking the part

Your dress should also reflect your seniority in an organization. A recruitment consultant once told me that to get promotion you need to dress for the job you want. In other words, you need to look the part, be that one or more rungs higher up the ladder than you currently are. The worst thing you can do is dress one rung lower. If you do get that promotion, you should immediately reassess your clothes and 'trade up'. Looking like a secretary when you have just become an executive is a bad idea.

Joining the culture club

There is also the culture of the company to think about. Every company has its own culture that covers what is acceptable in terms of behaviour, working patterns and dress. For example, there could be two firms, both manufacturing identical widgets, but one might have a dress-down culture, while to be seen without a tie at the other is a disciplinary offence. Before you start work for a new company, check out what goes and what doesn't. Arrange an informal drink with some of your new colleagues and scrutinize their clothes. Are the men wearing ties? Is anyone in jeans?

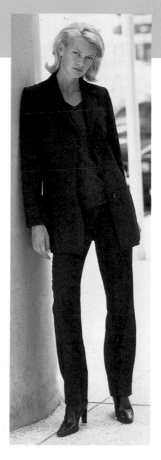

But we're getting ahead of ourselves. You haven't got that job yet. And you won't get it if you commit any of the following sins:

viewers will expect you to be in a suit. It is a compliment to them and shows you are taking the interview seriously.

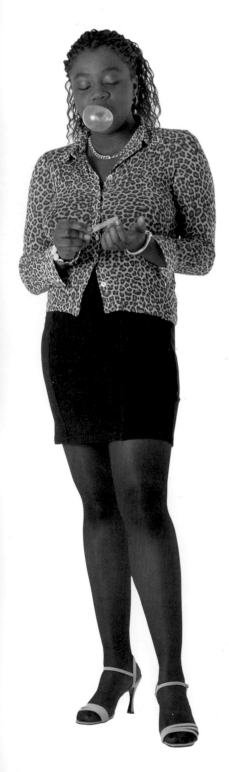

WHAT NOT TO WEAR TO A JOB INTERVIEW

jeans
shorts
anything see-through
pelmet skirt
leather and PVC
fishnet stockings
boots
stilettos
pierced nose/belly button

THE PERFECT INTERVIEW OUTFIT

**dark jacket, single-
or double-breasted**
**a matching skirt, on the knee
or just above**
**plain blouse
or jersey body**
dark tights
black or brown shoes
matching belt and handbag

Basically, any clothing you could imagine wearing on a beach or in a nightclub you shouldn't wear for a job interview. Overly sexy clothing will project entirely the wrong impression of how you see yourself contributing to the firm. Jeans and shorts suggest you are slovenly. As for a pierced nose (or a pierced anything), this is a bad idea unless you're up for a job selling the *Big Issue*. Any sort of boot is best avoided, as are stilettos – too tarty.

The bad news is that you need an interview suit

The image you are trying to project at a job interview is smart and professional. This means an 'interview suit'. This might sound old-fashioned. After all, Richard Branson is pretty successful and you never see him in a suit. But I wonder if he wore one in the early days when he needed an overdraft from the bank? I reckon he did. It is only once you become a multi-millionaire that you can flout dress codes. On the way up it is just too big a risk. The exceptions to the interview-suit rule are creative professionals, such as those in advertising and magazine art direction. Otherwise inter-

If this seems dull, it's supposed to. You're not on a Paris catwalk. You want your clothes to be as inoffensive as possible. It is for this reason that I suggest a skirt rather than trouser suit. There are still some companies and professions, law for example, that are suspicious of women in trousers. I had a boss a few years ago who announced that no woman who wore trousers would get promotion. And he meant it. Men like him assume any female not in a skirt is either a dangerous feminist or a lesbian, or both, in which case can he watch and, frankly, you don't want to get into that conversation.

The suit should be made up of a jacket in plain black, navy or grey. The skirt should be straight and on the knee or just above it. No shorter. It's worth spending money on a good suit. A cheap jacket often looks it. If you are seriously short of cash and you have to buy an inexpensive suit, check the topstitching in good light in the shop to see it's not wonky and give it a jolly good press before putting it on. A better idea still is to spend on a jacket what you would have on a suit. The jacket can then be teamed with a cheaper skirt. Instead of a blouse, you could also economize by opting for a 'body'. Again, a cheap 'body' will

So slick. Crisp pinstripes give a business-like appearance.

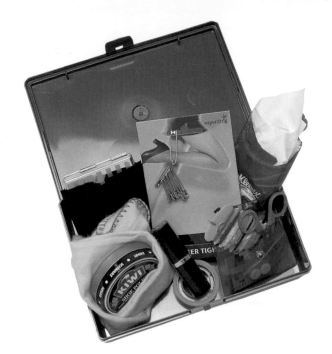

Ready for anything. Your emergency kit.

always look better than a cheap blouse.

One thing you can't really save money on is shoes. Real leather is essential. They should be a plain style. A low-heeled court shoe is best. Match these to your belt, if you're wearing one, and your handbag. Don't be tempted to try to dress up this admittedly dull outfit with 'interesting' tights or jewellery. Tights should be dark and plain, and jewellery should be kept to a minimum. Dangly earrings don't look professional. Bangles will rattle at the wrong moment.

Your outfit isn't finished yet, though. If you have long hair, tie it back with a simple fake tortoiseshell clip. Leave fancy bows for after-hours. If your hair is shorter, give yourself time before the interview to style it properly. Get it cut if it needs it. If you colour it, make sure your roots are done. Make-up is important: it makes you look 'put together'. Still, getting the amount right is tricky. Wear none and you won't

look polished. Wear too much and you'll look like a slapper. 'Subtle' should be your watchword. If you are not confident about applying it, choose a pale, pinkish lipstick, some mascara and just a little blusher, applied to the apple of your cheek, and leave it at that.

Your job interview survival kit

However well prepared you are for that interview, it's a good idea to take a few essentials with you. Then, if the worst happens – the button comes off your blouse, you ladder your tights – it's not a complete disaster. This lot should mean you're ready for anything:

1 Powder compact with mirror
2 Lipstick
3 Tissues
4 Spare pair of tights
5 Shoe polish and cloth (in case of nasty puddles)
6 Sewing kit
7 Sellotape (for sticking up hems quickly)
8 Half a dozen safety-pins in assorted sizes

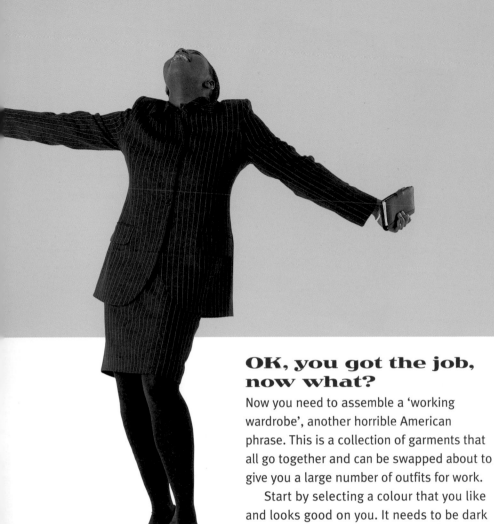

work with it. Good choices are black, navy, grey or brown. This is the colour of your suit, dress and the trousers. If you stick to the same colour for all these items then you immediately have three different outfits from only one jacket.

The suit should be as plain as possible. Fussy lapels, piping or other details will 'date' more quickly and can make something look tacky. The skirt should be straight and finish on or just above the knee. Buy wool if you can manage to. It will wear better than a synthetic. That said, the addition of Lycra to some fabrics is worth looking out for. It will prevent your suit creasing.

One tip: if your jacket, skirts or trousers have pockets which are sewn up when you buy them, do not unpick the stitching. I know it's a pain not to be able to carry things in your pockets, but if you can't put anything in them (including your hands), they won't sag. Your suit will look better for longer.

The trousers should be a classic straight-legged style. Remember, you're not making a fashion statement here. As for the dress, a plain shift shape is the most suitable for work. Make sure it has sleeves, though. Anything sleeveless does not look professional. Also, avoid floaty or see-though fabrics: they will make you look insubstantial.

Next, you need to select your accent colour. If you have more money, you could choose two accent colours, but one is enough. The accent colour should be one that looks good with your base colour. For example, if navy blue is your base, then bright red could be your accent. An accent doesn't have to be bright. A pale turquoise would work just as well as red. To choose an accent, take your suit with you when you're shopping for the rest of your wardrobe and experiment by holding blouses in different colours up against it. Your twinset, blouse and bodies should be in your accent colour.

OK, you got the job, now what?

Now you need to assemble a 'working wardrobe', another horrible American phrase. This is a collection of garments that all go together and can be swapped about to give you a large number of outfits for work.

Start by selecting a colour that you like and looks good on you. It needs to be dark and versatile. This is your base colour and everything else in your wardrobe has to

YOUR WORKING WARDROBE SHOPPING LIST

1 skirt suit

1 dress

1 twinset

1 pair trousers

2 bodies

1 blouse

1 mac/coat

2 pairs shoes

1 belt

1 handbag

3 pairs black opaque tights

It's up to you what proportion of your working wardrobe is in your base colour and what is in your accent. The more you choose in the base, the greater flexibility you will have. When it comes to shoes, belt and handbag, stick to black or brown and make sure they all match. The shoes should be low-heeled courts and the belt plain – no fancy buckles. The only other things you need are a coat in the base colour (if in doubt, go for a classic trench), some jewellery (a single string of pearls, a plain brooch and discreet earrings) and tights, which should be black and opaque. These are more expensive than sheers but don't ladder, so they last longer.

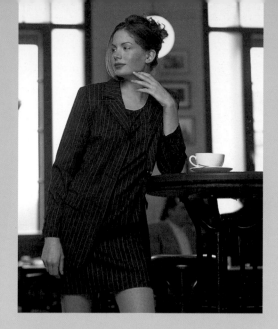

mere and from polyester to silk. Hopefully your salary will increase too so that you can afford to do this.

Once you have this basic collection of clothes, you can add to them as you earn more money. You can add a short pleated skirt, a pair of wide trousers, a long wrap-over skirt or another jacket. You can even add another base colour, if you like. Just remember to make sure that everything still goes together.

How to get a promotion

I have already mentioned dressing the part for the job you want, but how do you do that? Start by looking at the senior women in your company. Analyse the way they dress and copy it. You want to be one of them, so dress like one of them.

If there are no senior women, you'll have to improvise. Remember that saying, 'You have to speculate to accumulate'? Well, it holds true for office wear. You need to spend some money on your clothes. You can cheat a little, swap the buttons on a chain-store suit for expensive ones, drape a designer scarf over a bog standard twinset, that sort of thing. But if you're really serious about moving up, your clothes have to point the way. As you rise up in a company you need to spend more on the basics. You need to go from wool to cash-

Great! You're getting older and you've got to spend more on clothes

The other bit of bad news is that as you get older, you need to spend more. In part, this is because your girth is likely to increase and you won't be able to get yourself into cheaper, more skimpily cut clothes. But it is also a question of projecting the right image. Age equals gravitas and gravitas, I'm afraid, equals more expensive clothes. As a general rule, every 10 years you should double what you spend on an office outfit.

All women, whatever their age, need to think about the clothes they wear for work. It's about getting a professional polish. So, keep upgrading as and when you can. If you can afford it, have your hair professionally coloured rather than doing it yourself at home. It will look neater. Have a manicure, or give yourself one. If all this sounds like a job in itself, take heart. More and more of us are working from home. In a few years' time the 'working wardrobe' may be defunct. In the meantime, take off that suit when you get home from work and pour yourself a large drink. You deserve it.

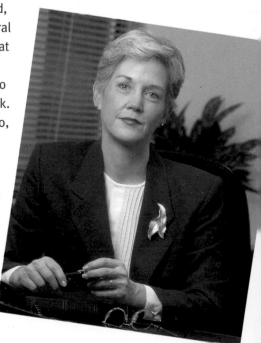

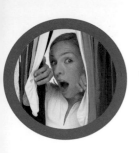

Rifle through the underwear drawer of almost any woman in Britain and you are sure to find two things: a pair of Marks and Spencer cotton briefs and a pair of black opaque tights.

Why a pair of black opaque tights
really is a girl's best friend

A woman might have had her cotton pants for decades, but her black tights are likely to be no more than five years old.

Still, they have roughly the same effect on her psyche. When a woman puts on her comfy knickers and her comfy tights she feels at peace. She feels safe, secure and ready to face the world.

It is only 10 years ago that opaque tights first arrived on the market. Before that tights were either sheer – remember micromesh? – or they weren't, in which case they were called support tights and only those with varicose veins wore them. There were woolly tights that little girls and librarians wore, but they went saggy round the knees and you had to darn the holes in them. Then black opaques were invented and changed everything.

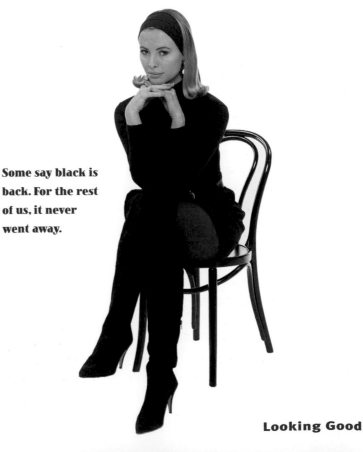

Some say black is back. For the rest of us, it never went away.

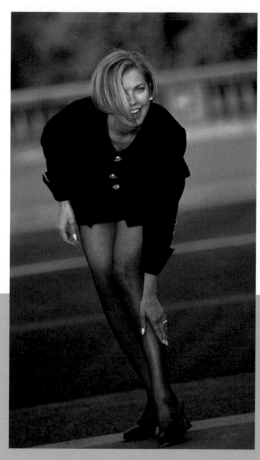

THREE GREAT THINGS ABOUT OPAQUES

1 THEY MAKE YOUR LEGS LOOK SLIMMER **2** YOU CAN WEAR A REALLY SHORT SKIRT WITH THEM AND YOU DON'T LOOK CHEAP **3** THEY DON'T LADDER

Stay in the dark. Funereal shades flatter any leg.

When designers first started putting opaques on the catwalk, they did it as a fashion statement. But that's not why women bought and continue to buy them in their thousands. We buy them because we know they make our legs look better – longer, slimmer, better. Sheer black tights perform the same vital function. The difference is that you see your skin through sheer tights. This makes them inherently sexy, which is fine for a night out, not so good for a staid office. Black opaques are asexual, which is why men hate them and women love them.

The thickness of opaques is crucial. You might be wearing only a thin knitted layer, but you feel covered up. They represent a vital barrier between you and the outside world. This is what makes them so brilliant with a short skirt. You don't feel so self conscious about showing your legs as you would in sheers. Plus, you can haul them on really fast in the morning without fearing you'll ladder them. Another major boon.

Which opaque is best?

There is now an almost infinite choice of opaque tights. However, some tights that call themselves opaque aren't. You need to buy at least 40 denier, preferably 70 denier, to get a sufficiently dense effect. Also, watch the finish. The most flattering styles are matt, not shiny. Lycra is pretty much an essential prerequisite if you don't want wrinkling at the knees and makes the tights much more comfortable. Choose those without Lycra and you can feel like you've had tight bandages tied round your legs. The addition of Tactel, a fibre that gives a silky texture, also improves the way they feel when on.

One of the greatest advances in tights during the last five years has been the introduction of a body-shaping element. You can now buy opaque tights that slim the waist, bottom and thighs. They are, admittedly, a bit more of a struggle to get on, but they're worth it.

Sheer seduction. Dustin Hoffman graduates from hosiery college.

Is there life beyond the black opaque?

The fashion world would like us to think so. They have been trying to tell us that black opaques are 'out' for at least four years. They tried pushing brown opaques for a while, then went to the opposite extreme and opted for natural-coloured tights. That didn't work. (Too many memories of the '70s for most of us.) Now they've settled on pastels. Can they really think that this bodes well for their profits? Who exactly wants mauve legs?

Still, let's be honest. You can't wear your opaques 12 months of the year, however much you love them. You'd look ridiculous and feel uncomfortable. There comes a point, usually some time in July, when you know you have to put aside your thick opaques for something lighter and cooler. It's a traumatic moment, a bit like the first time you put on a sleeveless summer dress. You get a heck of a shock at what your body really looks like. But it has to be done.

When looking for an alternative to the black opaque, bear the following in mind:

The need for novelty abounds. Manufacturers might want to ring the changes, but you don't have to.

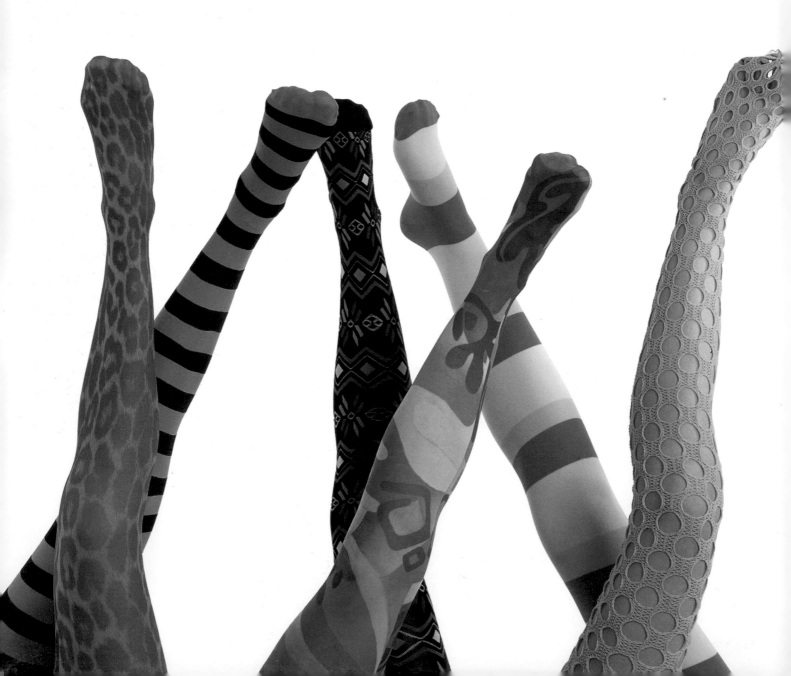

1
PATTERNED TIGHTS MAKE YOUR LEGS LOOK FAT

There are no two ways about it: tartan, spots, hoops, flowers – almost any print – will make you look hefty.

It almost makes you feel sorry for hosiery manufacturers. They must get so fed up of churning out boring black. 'Ooh, yes,' says one tights-maker to another, 'let's go wild and try a floral design this year.' Trouble is, we don't want floral tights. They might look OK on a catwalk, but on the average short, sturdy pair of legs patterned tights just look awful.

The exception to this rule is self-patterned, or textured, tights. Because they are all one colour, the pattern having been provided by different stitches, they are almost like plain tights. This makes them much more flattering .

The most long-running of self-patterns is lace. It can look good as long as the rest of the outfit is simple. Then again, too many frills and a bit too much jewellery and you could end up looking like Madonna when she was in her 'Like a Virgin' phase.

2
COLOURED TIGHTS MAKE YOU LOOK PECULIAR

My mother (yes, it's her again) has drawers full of tights in every colour ever made. When I was a child, I particularly dreaded the orange ones. She would pick me up from school looking like a human clementine. The lime ones weren't up to much either. The thing is that coloured tights, even if you match them exactly to your outfit (as my mother did), don't look natural. We do not have fuchsia legs – or hopefully we don't. Nor do we have turquoise or puce limbs.

Not all coloured tights are bad news. If they are dark, they can work. Chocolate brown, burgundy, bottle green or navy are all acceptable. Indeed, just slinging on black tights with a navy skirt looks lackadaisical.

Matching navy tights to a navy outfit, brown to brown and green to green looks classy and, so long as the hue is a deep one, they won't inflate your legs as much as brights.

3
AMERICANS NEVER HAD TANS LIKE THESE

Remember when natural tights were called 'American tan'? Most women in the '60s and '70s, never having crossed the Atlantic, weren't aware that American women didn't actually have tans the colour of the tights. We just assumed it was weBrits who were pasty. The truth is, of course, that no one has ever had a tan that colour in the history of the world.

These days American tan tights are much improved. For a start they're called 'natural'. They're also much paler in colour and much sheerer, so they let some of your own leg colour show through. Like opaques, there is a choice between matt or shiny. The latter can look quite good for more dressed-up occasions.

OK, naturals are never going to make your legs look stick thin, but in a situation when you can't wear black sheers or opaques – under a floaty summer dress, for example – then a good natural is about the best option. What will help is wearing a cream or beige shoe to match your tights. This will make your legs look longer.

Pale and interesting? Only if you have twiglet limbs.

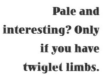
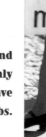

THE FIVE MOST DISGUSTING PAIRS OF TIGHTS OF ALL TIME

There are a few ideas that you shouldn't on any account even entertain:

5 COLOURED FISHNETS **4** HOOPED **3** STONE- OR BEIGE-COLOURED **2** WHITE WITH DIAMANTÉ BOWS AT THE BACK OF THE HEELS **1** TARTAN

Think top to toe

Hosiery designers might want to make a feature of their tights. It's in their interests. They might sell a few more pairs. However, tights are an accessory. They are there to complement the rest of an outfit, not dominate it.

So, before you buy any tights, consider what you are buying them to go with. Look at the colours in your wardrobe and purchase hosiery in a complementary hue.

YOUR BASIC HOSIERY SHOPPING LIST

3 pairs black opaques

1 pair navy opaques*

1 pair brown opaques*

6 pairs black sheers

1 pair natural sheers

*The brown and navy opaques are only applicable if you have brown and navy in your wardrobe. Otherwise stick to basic black. Remember, though, not to wear black tights with pale clothing – it looks naff.

If hosiery is that tricky, why can't I go bare legged?

At home, on holiday or in any casual social situation, of course you can go bare legged. In the workplace, however, tights are a must. No matter if the temperature is 90 degrees, a nude leg is unprofessional-looking. And if you think this is unfair, spare a thought for men in ties. They have to keep throttling themselves whatever the heat.

The only time you can get away without tights in a formal or work situation is if you're wearing trousers. A pair of cool linen trousers with sandals and no tights is perfectly acceptable. Don't be tempted to split the difference and wear pop socks though. When you sit down and cross your legs, you can always see a line where your pop socks pinch into your flesh. Tacky.

One last tip: tights can be very prone to picking up static electricity, which makes certain things cling to them. Making sure to fabric condition them after washing is one answer. But if you're on the way out of the door and you notice that your skirt is sticking to your thighs, a quick fix is to lick the palms of both hands and run them down your legs. A bit yucky, I know, but it works.

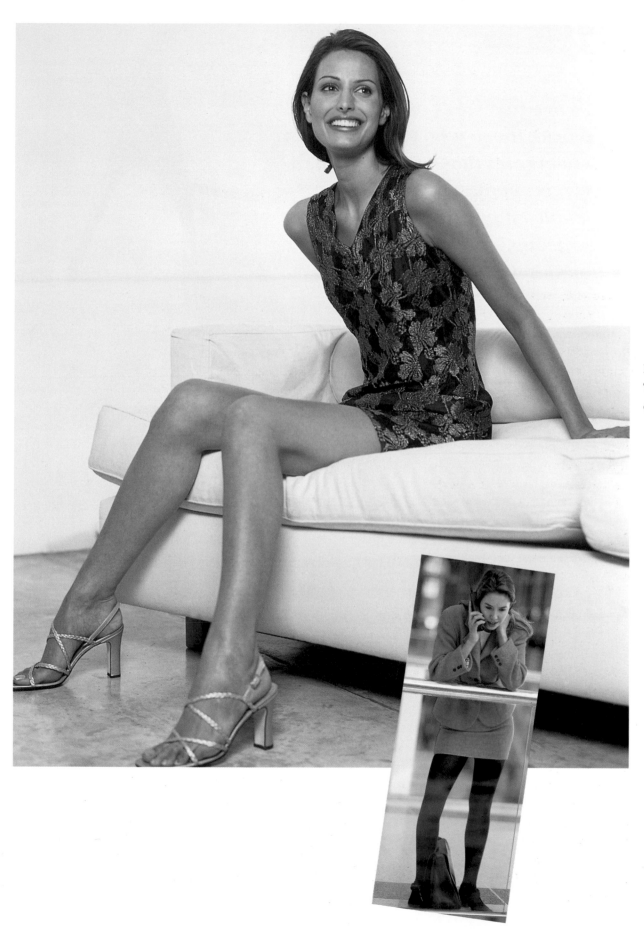

Dare to bare.
The right way to
go naked.

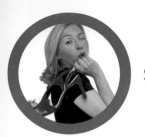
There are two sorts of women in the world: those who teeter about in high heels and those whose idea of heaven is slipping on a pair of Dr Scholls. If you are among the latter group, maybe you'd better skip this chapter.

To teeter or not to **teeter**

Film-star glamour. Big stars have always worn the biggest heels.

Dr Scholl sandals, healthy wonders though they may be, are not now, nor ever will be, staples of the fashionable wardrobe. Stick to them if you must, but don't ever expect to make the cover of *Vogue*.

I have to admit that I am biased. I belong to the high heels club. At only five feet tall, I am dangerously close to being munchkinesque. I need high heels. Actually, what I need is stilts, but I think people would stare at me in the street if I wore those. Still, it's not all about height. If I was five foot ten with legs like sticks of Brighton rock, I think I'd still want to wear heels. Short of hiring a Hollywood body double to walk about as you, 24 hours a day, putting on a pair of three-inch heels is the surest way to make yourself look instantly more attractive.

We're not talking sex here (we'll get to that in a minute). We're talking simple,

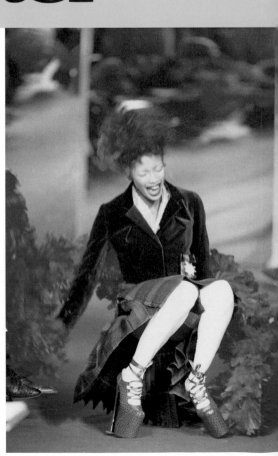

Sometimes you can go too far. Naomi comes a cropper.

HOW HIGH DO YOU GO?

This is pretty much up to you. Even a one-inch kitten heel can give you oomph. When deciding which heel height to go for, ask yourself these questions:

1 HOW GOOD AM I AT WALK-ING IN HIGH HEELS? **2** WHAT SURFACE WILL I BE WALKING ON? **3** HOW MUCH PAIN AM I WILLING TO PUT UP WITH?

physical fact. High heels make your legs look longer. Slip into spiky stilettos and even a girl with the calves of a cart horse can feel like Joanna Lumley.

The first time you put on a pair of high heels, you won't be able to walk in them, or maybe you will but you will look more like a duck than a human being. It takes practice to achieve poise. The key is to push your hips forward, your shoulders back and keep your chin up. Keep your spine straight and lean back slightly as you walk. Initially, this will feel both unnatural and precarious. But practice makes perfect.

Assessing the surface you are going to walk on is vital. Lino, marble or just wet pavement can be nightmares in high heels. Before venturing out, check the weather forecast and weigh up the odds of rain, snow, sleet or frost. If in doubt, lose an inch, otherwise that first step could take you straight to casualty.

A new hazard are those nobbly paving stones that have been installed at pelican crossings. They are intended as an aid to blind people and, as a former Girl Guide, I applaud that aim. However, HOWEVER, for high heel wearers they are a total pain in the backside. They must be approached with extreme caution, lest the uneven surface causes you to go over on one side of your foot.

DIY four-wheel drive

One way to lower the risk of serious injury is to treat the soles of a pair of new shoes before you wear them. At fashion shows, the bottom of every shoe is covered in masking tape, which is then scored with a pair of scissors to improve grip. Naomi Campbell's famous tumble aside, this does work, even if close up it's not very glamorous.

I prefer the pan-scourer trick. Take a pan scourer and rub it in circles across the shoe sole to create a roughened surface. It might break your heart to attack a brand new pair of shoes, but better that than break your neck in them. If you haven't got a pan scourer, a fork dragged across the bottom, as if you were fluffing up the mashed potato on top of a shepherd's pie is almost as good.

No pain no gain

This is a controversial topic. Why would, why should an intelligent woman in the '90s suffer for fashion? Were we discussing bubble skirts or any one of a thousand other hideous ideas that have come off the catwalk at one time or another, I would agree. But high heels make you look better, and I for one can stand a bit of discomfort to look better.

That said, you need to work out exactly how much discomfort you are going to have to put up with before you hand over your credit card in the shop. It is a fallacy that walking up and down a bit in a shoe shop gives you any idea at all how comfortable (or not) a pair of shoes is going to be. However gossamer soft those new stiletto sandals feel on a patch of Dolcis carpet, get them home and they are sure to be absolute agony.

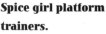

Spice girl platform trainers.

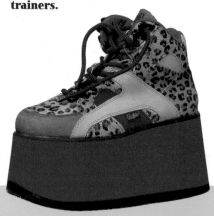

The pan-scourer trick...

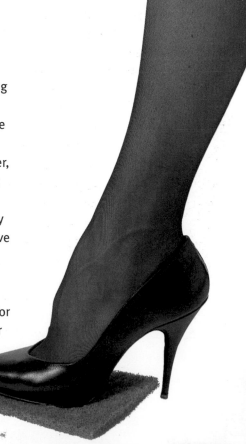

SO HOW DO I KNOW HOW UNCOMFORTABLE THEY'RE GOING TO BE?

You can get a pretty good idea from just looking at the shoe.
What you are looking for are six factors:

1 HEEL HEIGHT **2** HEEL WIDTH **3** HEEL ANGLE
4 STABILITY OF THE SHOE **5** WIDTH ACROSS THE BALL OF THE FOOT **6** SHOE SIZE

I was in a shoe shop once with a boyfriend, hobbling up and down in a pair of very high shoes. 'What do you think?' I foolishly asked my squeeze. 'Well, as long as they're comfortable' was his memorable reply. Comfortable! Was the man insane? They had four-inch heels. Of course they weren't comfortable.

Obviously, when you're talking about anything above a two-inch heel, there is a level of discomfort to be dealt with. And the higher the heel, the more painful the shoe will be, particularly if you intend wearing it for long periods. But it isn't just a matter of height. You also need to look at width. A wider heel spreads the weight of your body, even if only slightly, and also improves your balance.

Next, look at the angle of the heel. A slanted Cuban heel is, broadly speaking, more uncomfortable than a gently curving stiletto. Vertical and Louis heels can also be dodgy. The thing to watch out for in either case is that the heel is not set too far back. If it is, it will force all your body weight on to the ball of your foot, which can be agony.

Apart from the heel itself, the ball of the foot is the other crucial area to study. It is this that takes the bulk of your weight. If the section of the shoe over the arch and toes is narrow and you have to squish your toes to get into it, then you are asking for trouble. Winkle-pickers are very bad news indeed. Look for shoes that feel roomy, but are not loose.

Improving the stability of shoes will make them feel more comfortable and make your calves and ankles less tired. So try to find shoes with plenty of 'body' to them. By that, I mean avoid sandals with only a couple of strips of leather holding the shoe on. Look for high-heeled court shoes or those with ankle straps. Anything that makes them feel sturdier. If you choose a very cut-away style, you might have to grip with your toes to keep them on, which will cause claw feet.

Move over Imelda Marcos. A girl can never have too many pairs of shoes.

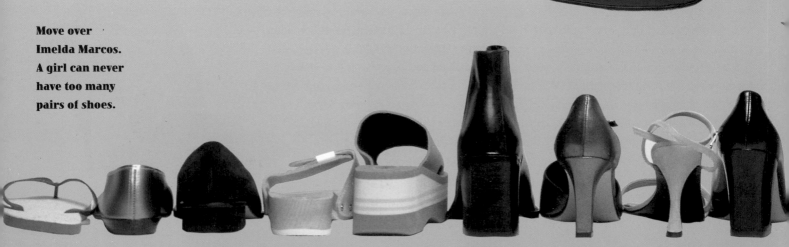

I just need to wear them in a bit

If you find yourself saying this, then do not buy those shoes. You are not wearing them in, you are wearing your feet in. That said, all new shoes have sharp edges, particularly inside, that rub your feet. One tip is to take an emery board and file down any seams or edges that stick up inside the shoes before you wear them. As an extra precaution, on their first outing, take a few plasters with you, just in case you feel your feet getting sore.

Are there any naff high heels?

Of course there are. They are called white stilettos. On the Continent they don't see anything wrong with white stilettos. Walk up the Via Della Spiga, Milan's answer to Bond Street, and you see loads of women in white stilettos. But they're also wearing sunglasses with horrible gold fiddly bits on the side and too much fake tan, so they're not really in a position to act as fashion icons, are they?

In Britain the white stiletto will never escape its Essex girl tag. So if you're tempted, resist. The only possible occasions when white shoes are OK are when it's very, very hot and at a wedding. Hot weather makes white strappy sandals just about acceptable, so long as they are very flimsy with as few straps and as much foot

on display as possible. White bridal shoes are all right, but they should be made of silk, not leather.

In any case, white shoes should never, never be accompanied by the following:

1   An ankle chain.
2   An ankle tattoo of a swallow, rose or dolphin.
3   White stirrup trousers.
4   Anything made from snow-wash denim.

Other really nasty high heels

Coloured high heels are a problem, except for in the evening. After six o'clock you can get away with almost anything. During the day, however, heels in any colour except black, navy or brown can look tarty. If in doubt, don't.

Also, high heels with things on are best avoided. Bows on the front of shoes or, worse, the backs of heels are horrible. Fancy topstitching or contrast 'lashing', gold studs, diamante or fancy buckles are all no-nos.

High-heeled boots are a tricky area. In theory they are fine. In practice they invariably look like they have stepped straight from the window of an Anne Summers shop. High-heeled cowboy boots, with or without Navajo-style, turquoise-effect jewelling and tassels, are best kept for the line dancing class.

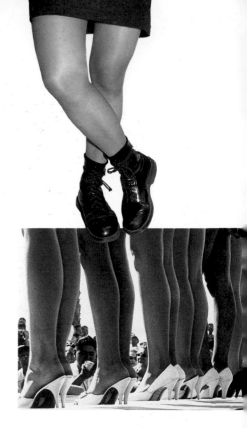

Footwear faux pas: Doctor Marten boots and white stilettos.

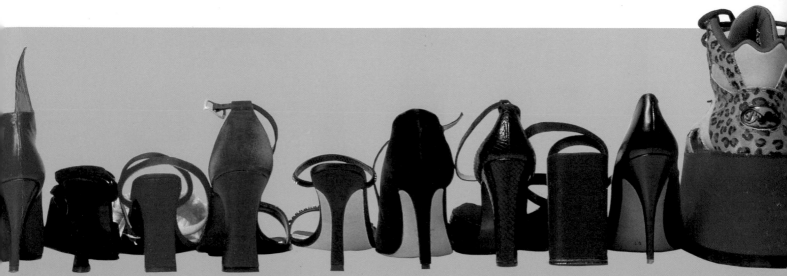

What about flats?

Putting aside my natural aversion to flats, I will admit there are good flatties and bad flatties.

Flat shoes, as far as shoe designers are concerned anyway, are dull. The desire to tart them up a bit, get creative, add some interest, some novelty, is ever-present. But do not succumb. Remember, shoes are accessories. They always look better if they are kept plain, otherwise the different parts of your outfit can begin competing with each other. This is known as Sue Pollard syndrome and should be avoided at all costs.

The best flatties are the classics – simple, honest designs that look classy and up-market. For work, loafers or lace-up brogues in black or brown leather will look good with trousers. With a skirt, you're better off with ballet pumps, again in black or brown, plus perhaps navy or red. Wear brogues with a skirt and you are liable to look just a tad butch.

More casual occasions demand old-fashioned plimsolls – the cotton lace-up type. Please don't buy fancy espadrilles. They always look wrong. Navy, white or

GOOD FLATTIES

LOAFERS • BROGUES • OLD-FASHIONED PLIMSOLLS
• FLIP-FLOPS • ROMAN SANDALS • BALLET PUMPS

BAD FLATTIES

Dr Scholl Sandals • TRAINERS
• GOLD ESPADRILLES

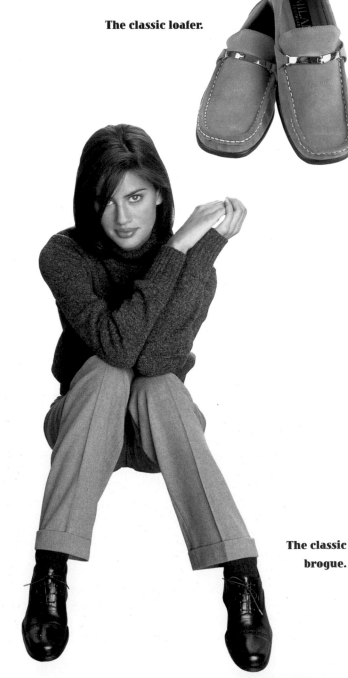

The classic loafer.

Flatties don't have to be dull.

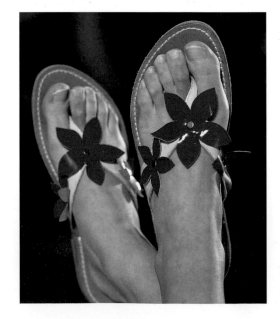

The classic brogue.

SHOE ESSENTIALS

If you want to start from scratch and build up a versatile collection of shoes, get yourself the following:

1 PAIR BLACK COURT SHOES WITH TWO-AND-A-HALF-INCH HEELS • 1 PAIR BROWN COURT SHOES WITH TWO-AND-A-HALF-INCH HEELS • 1 PAIR BLACK STILETTOS WITH THREE- TO FOUR-INCH HEELS, POSSIBLY SLING-BACKS • 1 PAIR FLAT BROWN LACE-UP BROGUES • 1 PAIR FLAT BROWN LEATHER SANDALS • 1 PAIR OLD-FASHIONED NAVY PLIMSOLLS

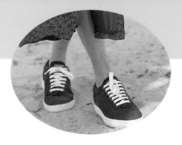 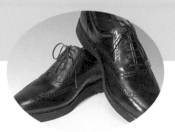 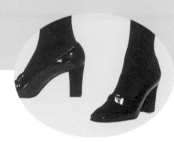

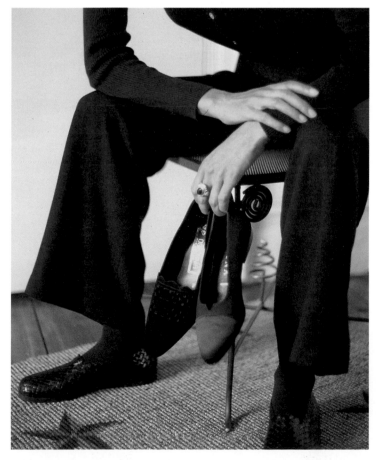

beige plimsolls are far more stylish, as well as being cheap. For really hot weather, or for a holiday, tan leather roman sandals and basic black flip-flops (eschew neons) are chic and fun.

I know I have a bit of an obsession about trainers, but I hate them, except when worn for sport. If you find them easy and comfortable to wear, fine. But they really do murder any outfit. Try to wear something else.

Now you know what should be your basics. You can add anything else you want. But with just these shoes, you should have everything you need.

Comfort and elegance can go together.

How much do I have to spend?

Cheap shoes are not a good idea. Anything that's not made of leather will make your feet perspire. That said, you can economize on summer shoes. Plastic sandals are fine as your foot can 'breathe'.

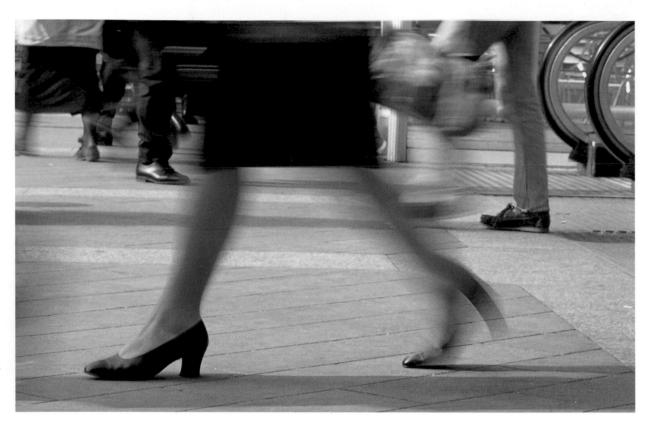

Which shoe with which outfit?

Basic courts: practical but dull.

You can pack your wardrobe with more designer shoes than Imelda Marcos and still look a mess if you team the wrong shoe with the wrong outfit. What complicates things is that whereas one year to wear heels with trousers is the height of fashion, the next it is fashion death.

As a general rule, mannish clothes look better with mannish shoes. So trousers, jeans, trouser suits will appear more stylish with a flat brogue than a stiletto. If you need the height, an ankle boot with a small heel will also look good.

Thicker heels don't have to be clumpy.

When it comes to dresses, an enduring teenage fashion is to team these with tough boots and thick socks. On Kate Winslett this looks ravishing. Anyone else should think twice. A 'ladylike' – what a horrible word – shoe rather than an ankle boot will jar less and be kinder to your legs.

As for high heels, these should rise at night. During the day, two or three inches is the norm. After dark is when you get out your real spikes. Sling-backs and peep-toed styles are also far more in keeping with a little black dress than an office suit.

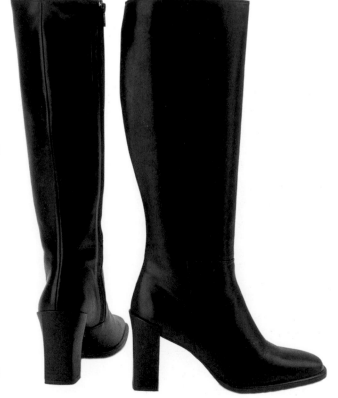

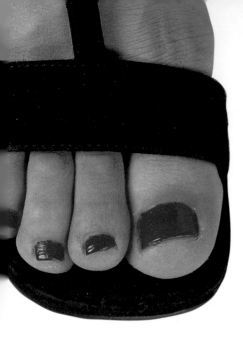

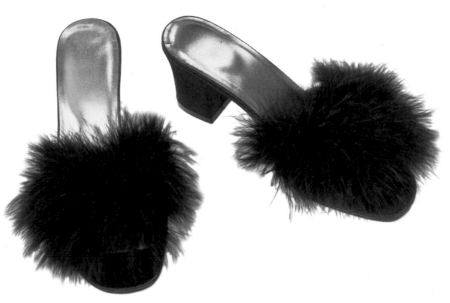

Just the thing for a quiet night in. Fluffy film-star mules.

Shoes and seduction

There is no doubt that if you want a direct line to the part of a man's brain labelled L for lust, then shoes are one way to do it. Subtler than putting on a crotch-length mini or a plunge-necked tee-shirt, the right shoes are nevertheless highly erotic.

We're not talking just about a few sad men in macs here. For a large slice of men, even the majority perhaps, shoes are enormously sexy. And the more feminine the shoes, the sexier they are. Broadly speaking, the more your shoes differ from a style he might wear, the more attractive he will find them, and you.

Stilettos are the obvious sexy shoe. But they can be too obvious. Better to steer clear of white or red. Wear a pair of white stilettos and he'll assume all he has to do is pour a couple of lager and limes down you and you're his for the night. Wear red and he won't even bother with the drinks. He's liable to spreadeagle himself over his

Think spiky...

car on the way to the wine bar and yell 'Take me, take me now!'

Black is by far the sexiest colour for a stiletto. Shiny black patent is racier still. If you really want to be adventurous, there is always the shiny black stiletto boot, but then the kind of man you'll pick up in those will probably want to be led around your kitchen on all fours on a leash. (Still, if he wouldn't mind putting a J-cloth and a bit of Jiff round while he's there, he could come in useful.)

Toe cleavage

For those unfamiliar with this term, toe cleavage refers to the cracks between your toes. Reminiscent of breast cleavage, only naughtier – Chinese men used to... well perhaps we won't go into that – toe cleavage is a major male turn-on. If you really want to raise the temperature on a date, wear a pair of shoes cut away at the front to reveal your toe cleavage. I guarantee he'll be fanning himself with his napkin by dessert.

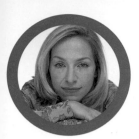

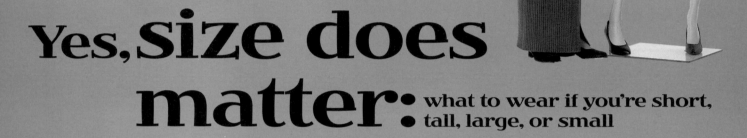

Have you ever stood next to a shop dummy? Next time you're in a shop, give it a try. It's very instructive.

Yes, size does matter: what to wear if you're short, tall, large, or small

The first thing you'll notice is how tall a shop dummy is compared to you. 'Her' hips will be where your waist is, for example. But, it isn't just that 'she' is tall. She is also very thin. Those hips will be about the width of one of your thighs, that waist as wide as your neck. In fact, the more you look, the more you will realize how skew-whiff 'her' proportions are. 'Her' arms, legs and neck will be grossly elongated, while her body is strangely shortened. It's as if the mannequin-makers had taken a normal woman, made an effigy of her in bubblegum and then just stretched selective bits.

And that, of course, is exactly what does happen when they make shop dummies. Only worse. They take a model – hardly a normal female to begin with – and then exaggerate her features. Her breasts become perkier, her buttocks more pert, her arms are made skinnier and her legs just a few inches longer. The result is a travesty of

the truth of the way you or I look. And yet it stands staring from every shop window.

Supermodels are often blamed for making the rest of us feel depressed about our appearance. Certainly, a constant diet of fashion shown on supermodels is not the most cheerful experience. (This is why *Looking Good* operates a partial supermodel ban in its programmes.) But at least Kate & Co. are human, sort of. Shop dummies are unreal, literally.

The reason I say you should stand next to a shop dummy is so that you realize this – so that you understand just how unreal mannequins are. Further, it's so that you should never again go through that thing where you see something in a shop window looking gorgeous, then try it on and wonder why it looks so much worse on you. 'God, I must be a really odd shape,' you think. Stand next to that dummy and you'll realize once and for all.

IT'S NOT YOU. IT'S 'HER' THAT'S WEIRD.

No one looks like shop dummies, not even supermodels. Instead, we are all a bit smaller, a bit taller, we have thicker waists, flatter chests, shorter legs, longer arms, etc. We are all different. Except we all want the same thing: to be able to put clothes on in the morning and not feel like a total blimp. Yes, it probably is easier to avoid blimpdom if you're Helena Christensen. But there we are.

As my grandmother always said: 'Life isn't fair.' The job of this chapter is to even the odds up a little in your favour. If you're short, tall, very skinny or wear a size 18 or over, there are particular tricks of the fashion trade that can help you make the best of your raw material.

in the kind of stuff available. Wallis, Next, Marks and Spencer, and Principles are among those who now cater to the more diminutive of stature. That said, there is a big problem with 'petite' lines. You have to be 'petite' to wear them.

Just because you are short it does not mean that you are 'petite'. When I was a size 18, I had a 40-inch bust and similar hips. I was not remotely 'petite'. Still, manufacturers assume that every woman under five foot three looks like Kylie Minogue. We don't. We look like everyone else, only we are shorter waisted and have abbreviated arms and legs.

While 'petite' manufacturers continue to act like ostriches when presented with this information, we, the customers, have to make do with what is available both in 'petite' lines and clothes for 'normal' people. In fact, it's often better to look elsewhere – petite lines have a habit of lagging six months behind everything else fashionwise.

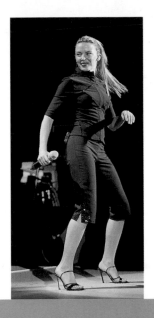

Pedal pushers: strictly for the long-legged.

All the best things come in small packages

If you're five foot three or under (as I am), you'll be very fed up of hearing that one. All the best things might come in small packages, but if you are one of those small packages, it's not much fun trying to wrap yourself in clothes. Hands disappear up sleeves, legs trail acres of useless trouser fabric, mini skirts become maxis, long jackets turn into coats.

The petite fallacy

Whenever a short person whinges about the difficulty of finding clothes to fit, she is pointed in the direction of 'petite' lines. 'Look,' say the experts, 'there is lots of choice for short a*** like you now.' Certainly, there has been an improvement

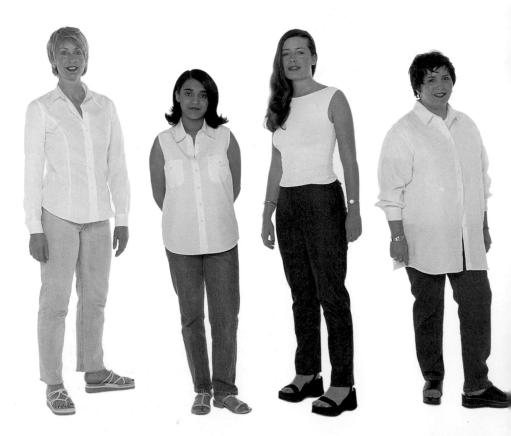

WHAT NOT TO WEAR IF YOU DON'T WANT TO LOOK LIKE YOU'VE BEEN HAMMERED INTO THE GROUND

baggy jumpers

long full skirts

jackets longer than your bottom

wide-shouldered jackets

swing coats

lampshade ballgowns

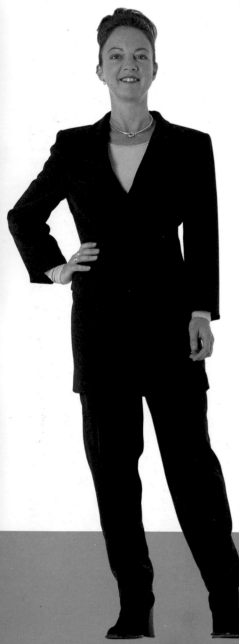

Long and lean trouser suit.

Remember this?
Me having my
hair chopped by
Anthony
Yacomini on
Looking Good.

The key if you are short is to avoid swamping yourself. Loose layers might feel comfortable, especially if you've put on a few pounds and you're trying to hide it, but they will make you look much stumpier. Long lengths, be they a jacket that drops to mid-thigh or an ankle-skimming skirt, will have the same effect.

Speaking as someone who thought she'd grow up to lounge languidly on a chaise longue, pipe-cleaner limbs folded elegantly beneath her, but instead finds a toadstool and fishing rod are far more appropriate, I know how frustrating it is to have to rule out whole looks just because of your height, or lack of it. However, put aside any notions of wafting about in Jemima Khan-ish loose layers. They just won't look good on you.

Likewise, mannish suits with shoulder-padded jackets can overpower you. If you do want to wear a jacket with shoulder pads, go for something with fairly discreet padding and be especially careful about 'doubling up'. This is what happens when you slip a shoulder-padded shirt under a shoulder-padded jacket and stick a shoulder-padded coat over the top. The result is that, like American footballers, your neck disappears. Swing coats and evening dresses with very full skirts are another hazard. They will make you look like a mushroom.

WHAT TO WEAR TO LOOK TALLER

fitted jackets

short skirts

narrow-legged trousers

shift dresses

three-quarter-length coats

high heels

To make yourself look taller and thinner, you need to streamline yourself. Jackets that nip in at the waist are great, if you've got the waist. If you haven't, go as fitted as you can and don't be tempted to let the length of the jacket drop too low. The hem should finish no longer than the top of your thighs, otherwise you will make your legs look even shorter.

To go with this jacket, choose a short skirt if you have good legs, or narrow-legged trousers. Again, you need to go as narrow as you can. If you have big legs any trouser will still be more flattering than a long skirt. Long skirts always risk turning short women into daleks.

A short shift dress and three-quarter-length coat continue the don't swamp yourself theme. Team these with tights and shoes that match to increase the overall impression of height. When in doubt, put on higher heels.

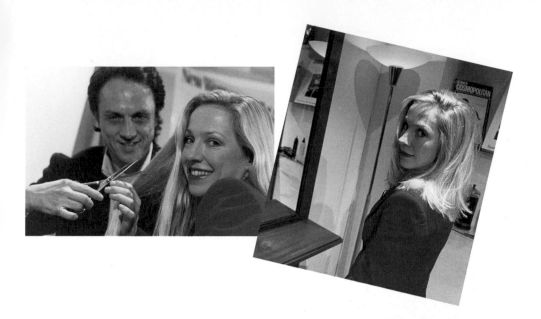

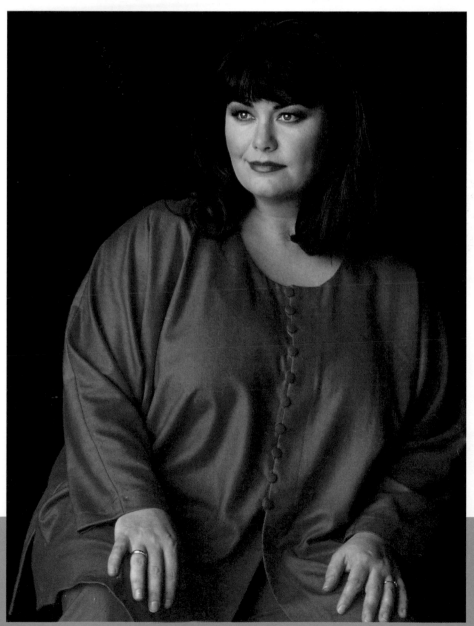

**Wonder woman.
Dawn French
proves larger
doesn't have to
mean dowdier.**

All change

If you are short, almost everything you buy
will have to be altered. You can do it yourself, but it's a hassle and you're likely to get
a more professional finish by letting the
professionals do it. The thing is, this costs
money, as much as £25 on top of the price
of a suit. Only, it doesn't have to.

I am not a great supporter of store
cards. I think they are just another way to
encourage all of us to run up debt. That
said, there is a real benefit to having some
store cards – a free alterations service. This
is a boon for short women. So next time
you're trying something on, ask an assistant if you can have it altered free. If you
can't, go elsewhere.

Going for the chop

As I discovered in the last series of *Looking
Good*, cutting your hair really can make you
look taller. Like so many women, I'd
become wedded to my long hair and was
really nervous about losing it. 'I'll never
date again,' I thought as the hairdresser
loomed over me with his scissors. However,
long hair on short women can get a bit
overwhelming and Rapunzel-like if you
don't watch it. Short or shoulder-length
hair really does suit shorter proportions
much better. Take the plunge. You won't
regret it. I haven't.

What's the weather like up there?

Jo Brand: a role model in more ways than one.

If short women get a hard time, tall women probably have it even worse. At least if you are small, you can take up the sleeves on a jacket or the hem on a pair of trousers. Tall women don't have this flexibility. If the extra fabric isn't there, it isn't there. They are reduced to having to order special length garments, always wear short styles or walk about like Michael Jackson.

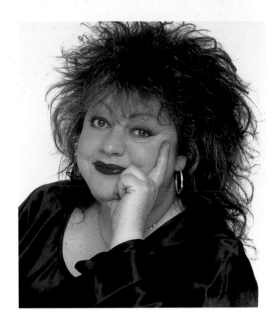

WHAT TO WEAR TO MAKE THE MOST OF YOUR HEIGHT

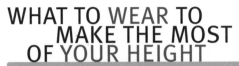

mini skirts
loose layers
cropped tops
wide trousers
long skirts
mid-thigh-length jackets
long, sweeping coats
knee boots

If you are tall, you are the only woman who will ever look good in an ankle-length greatcoat. For that alone you should give fervent thanks. While shorties like me have to shuffle around in car coats, you can sweep about being dramatic. Long skirts, especially if they are slit, will look fantastic on you, as will longer jackets and loose tunic-style tops worn over wide trousers.

But it's not just long lengths that suit tall women – mini-skirts can look sensational, especially worn with knee boots. Indeed, if you want to lessen the effect of your height, going for short clothes is one way to do it. Cutting up your body by wearing a cropped top with a mini and knee boots is very effective.

Make-up

Hair and make-up are really important if you are a tall woman. You need to emphasize your femininity. This doesn't mean apologizing for your height – it's just reminding people that you are all woman. I learned this from a friend of mine who is six foot two in her bare feet. She always looked great until she had her hair cut. She had a crop and the first time I saw her I thought: 'Who is that man?' Evidently, so did a lot of others. My friend swiftly took to wearing bright lipstick and started growing her hair back.

Stealing from his wardrobe

Another good thing about being tall is that you can steal stuff from your partner's wardrobe. Since menswear is invariably better made and often cheaper than womenswear, it also pays to buy in the men's department. Remember though, tee-shirts and sweaters are OK; whole suits and you look like Grace Jones.

When's the baby due?

We've covered how to dress to make yourself look slimmer in the 'Fat Days' chapter

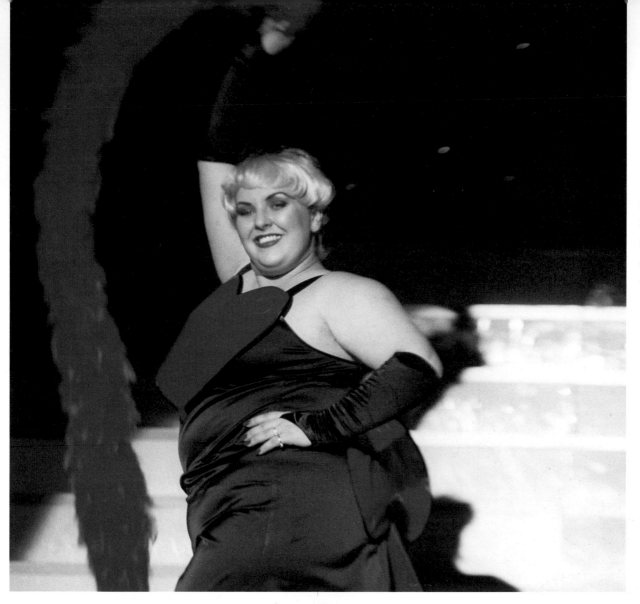

on page 22.
However, if you find people asking you when the baby's due, I have one more tip for you. Tell them to get a life and get on with your own.

Skinny Lizzy

I can't say I have a great deal of sympathy with people who complain that they can't put on weight. 'Oh, I just forget to eat,' they always say. Yeah, right. The rest of us forget to eat all the time. Yesterday I forgot to eat for maybe one millisecond. However, I will overcome my natural instinct to give skinny girls a good slap and try to be empathetic.

If you would like to look as if you have a few more curves, the first step is to throw out anything in your wardrobe that is stretchy and clingy. Nothing looks worse than a garment that is supposed to cling but actually bags. Flimsy, floaty dresses that hint at the body beneath are going to suit you much better.

Next, look for garments with some detail on, both to bulk you out and distract attention from coat-hanger collar bones or bony legs. Tops with a ruched or laced front will give the impression of a cleavage. Skirts that are gathered into the waist or pleated will pad thin hips. Layers of knitwear will add bulk all over.

All this advice flies in the face of everything I know about clothes, but then I, like practically every other woman I've ever met, spend my life trying to look slimmer, not fatter. If you're one of the lucky skinny ones, spare a thought for the rest of us.

Big and bold. If you wear a larger size, don't apologize for it – enjoy yourself.

Yes, tall girls have problems buying clothes too (or so I am told).

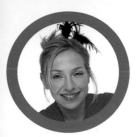

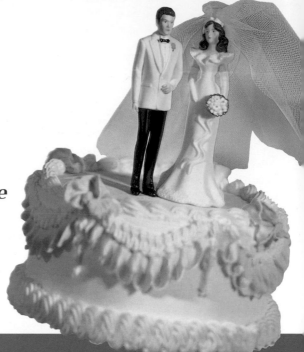

There cannot be an occasion more likely to cause a fashion disaster than a wedding. Even if you're not the bride, the sartorial performance pressure is huge.

Weddings, christenings and other clothes crises

There you are with your family, your friends, possibly a few ex-lovers and their new partners. You're all gathered together, jealousies and insecurities brought gently to simmering point by copious amounts of alcohol. Add to this the fact that you're wearing a new pair of shoes and rain has just ruined your hugely expensive designer hat and, frankly, it's a wonder more wedding guests don't come to blows over the smoked salmon pinwheels.

The British both love and hate formal occasions, not just weddings but christenings, bar mitzvahs, any chance to put on a posh frock in fact. We love them because they give us a chance to engage in our favourite pastime: keeping up with the Joneses. Conversation at the reception will be almost entirely made up of speculation as to the cost per plate of the buffet and an estimate of the length of the bride's train. We hate these occasions for the

Leg of mutton sleeves: don't do it.

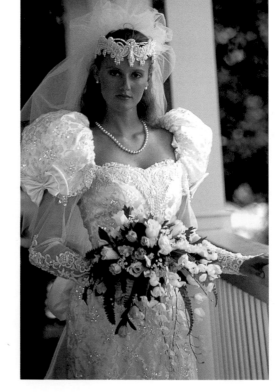

A FEW BASIC RULES FIRST:

PLAN AHEAD

Outfits for formal occasions cannot be thrown together. It is not just your reputation at stake here – you're dealing with family pride. And any mistakes aren't going to go away. They will live on in family albums for decades, so give it some thought.

CONSULT OTHERS

Before deciding what to wear, you should consult the other female members of your family to ensure your outfit is not going to clash, or, worse, they have not bought exactly the same thing.

CONSIDER THE HIERARCHY

Other than the bride, the mother of the bride's outfit takes precedence. It is good manners, therefore, not to upstage her by wearing a brighter colour than her. (Of course, if you do want to upstage her...) Find out what she's wearing and bear it in mind. The same goes for the mother of a baby at a christening or the mother of a boy at a bar mitzvah.

THINK ABOUT WHERE YOU WILL BE

If the reception is to be held inside, the choice is easy. You simply need an outfit that isn't too hot. If, however, the reception is in a marquee set up in a garden, you will need a jacket or wrap of some kind in case it gets chilly. Also, don't wear spiky heels. They will sink into the grass.

same reason – we hate the pressure of being judged.

Still, there's no getting out of them. So how do you pass muster in front of even the most demanding relatives?

Now, down to specifics.

Meringue skirt: who needs more bulk around their bottom?

Here comes the bride, all fat and wide

Well, hopefully not actually. The thing is, white is not the most slimming colour and when you start adding frills and flounces it could turn Jodie Kidd into Big Bertha. Yes, this is your big chance to look like the princess out of a fairy tale, but beware of ending up looking like the fairy on top of a Christmas tree.

Which style of dress is right for you?

You can find this out only by trying on lots and lots. However, there are a few guidelines. Dresses with big skirts are always less flattering than those with a more streamlined shape. Big puff sleeves, for example, are difficult to carry off unless you have a long neck, while anything high-necked will make a large bust look matronly.

THE THREE MOST UNFLATTERING WEDDING DRESS DESIGNS

1 TIERED LAMPSHADE DRESS

2 PUFF-SLEEVED FAIRY-QUEEN DRESS

3 ANYTHING WITH A CONTRAST CUMMERBUND

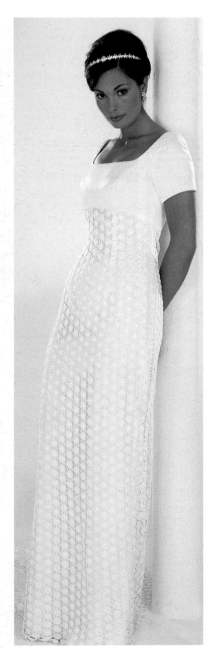

Coolly elegant, and you get to cover your upper arms too!

Going for a slightly retro look is a good way of avoiding Christmas fairy syndrome. You get the romance without the acres of frills. A '20s flapper dress design is especially flattering because it skims the body. Be careful if you have a full bust, though. It could make you look like a barrel on legs.

A more '30s-style slip dress, as worn by Caroline Besset when she married John F. Kennedy Junior, is good if you want something even simpler. If you need to wear a bra, it can cause problems though. Those little shoe-string straps aren't going to hide anything. A strapless bra or corset-top hidden underneath are your best bets.

The '50s shift with flared train is a good idea if you are determined to have a real 'entrance frock'. From the front it looks straight. All the fullness is in the back and in the train, making it much more flattering than a standard lampshade.

Will they snigger if I walk down the aisle in white?

The days when you had to be a virgin to wear white are now long gone. This is fortunate, otherwise all the manufacturers of white wedding dress lace would be out of business by now. Even so, eyebrows will be raised if you are eight months pregnant and you insist on staggering down the aisle in snowy white satin.

An off-white dress is both safer and can look more expensive. Pure, glowing white can look a bit cheap and synthetic, whereas off white is more stylish and classy. If you are not marrying for the first time, already have children together, or are an older bride, ivory, cream or pearl are better choices. Or you could go for a pastel shade of blue, pink or yellow. The idea is to look fresh, but not to stretch credibility too far.

There has been a fashion over the last few years of wedding dresses in outrageous colours. If you want to get married in black, purple or lime green, go ahead. But just remember, if you go wild and wacky, you're going to have that wedding picture on your mantelpiece for a very long time.

Keeping it simple

If you are getting married in a register office, you should scale things back a bit. A huge white frock will look incongruous in municipal surroundings. However, this doesn't mean you can't have your dress of a lifetime. Why not wear a smart suit for the official bit, then change before the reception into your romantic dress? That way, you can have the pictures done with you looking gorgeous, but not feel an idiot trying to get eight petticoats through the door to the register office.

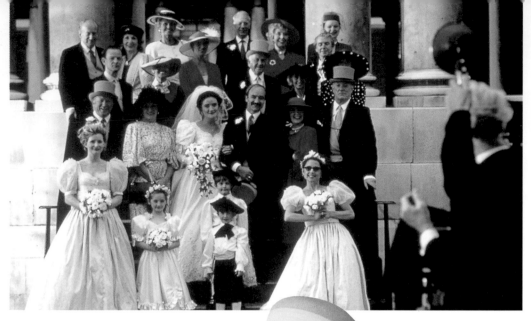

Four Weddings and a Funeral... or how the other half do it.

Taking the plunge or not

You might consider your cleavage to be your best feature, but it is probably one that is best kept under wraps on your wedding day. Remember, you're supposed to look sweet and unblemished – well, you're supposed to have a stab at it anyway. So don't wear a very plunging dress. If you have a full bust and want to avoid looking matronly in a high neck, have the front cut relatively low, but a sheer fabric added over the top to shield the congregation in the church from the full force of your bared bosoms.

Bridal finishing touches

It's wise to keep the dress as plain as possible because, as the bride, you're going to have a lot of bits and pieces to go with it. You will be holding a bouquet, possibly a hymn book or Bible as well. Then there is your veil, possibly a headdress, gloves, not to forget your wedding ring... Start adding fancy bits to your frock and you'll look like Little Bo Peep before you know it.

Right: For the racier bride a printed fabric, but still a slim shape.

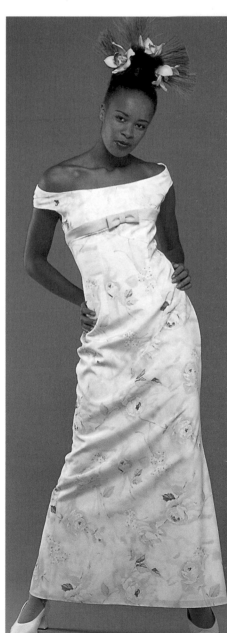

Left: You can't go wrong with a nippy little suit. Swap the skirt for trousers if your legs aren't up to it.

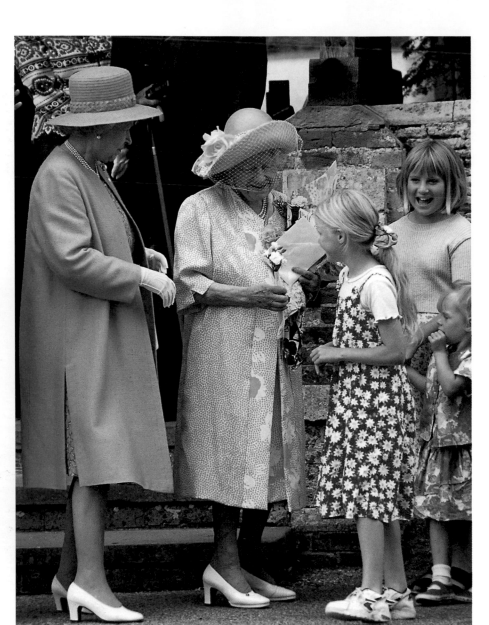

1

They choose a frock that looks good on the slim bridesmaid, without considering how it will look sized-up for the larger ones. The result is one ravishing attendant and three looking lumpy in floral frills.

2

They decide how they want their child bridesmaids to look first, then have matching dresses run up for the grown-ups. This means the little ones look sweet, while the bigger ones look stupid.

PLEASE AVOID

coral, mauve or mint green

floral prints

puff sleeves

contrast cummerbunds

Still, if you are a bridesmaid and you find yourself dressed in something you absolutely hate, keep calm and grit your teeth. Remember, it's for one day only and it's not your day, it's the bride's.

She's the nation's favourite grand-mother, but that doesn't mean you have to wear her hats.

The good brides-maid's dress guide

I've been a bridesmaid three times. Admittedly, I was less than ten on all three occasions. I still can't say I was a big fan of the outfits I had to wear. But then, the very act of accepting an invitation to be a bridesmaid is to give up any say in what you will be wearing.

Brides often make massive mistakes when deciding what to dress their brides-maids in. These mistakes usually fall into two categories:

How to dress the perfect guest

The little, nippy skirt suit is now the accepted uniform for guests invited to everything from a wedding to a 25th wedding anniversary. You could try a dress and jacket, but avoid anything droopy. You should look sharp and polished.

The best combination is a single-breasted jacket, fitted to just below the hip and a skirt on the knee or just above it. The shape of the skirt should be straight, A-line or pleated. You could substitute a trouser suit for the skirt suit. If you are larger, a jacket that skims the bottom and matching soft trousers cover a multitude of sins. Team with a simple silk tee-shirt, sheer tights and matching shoes.

GOOD COLOUR COMBINATIONS

navy and white/black and white
red and black
any bright colour, so long as you keep the outfit to just one colour

any pastel, so long as you keep the outfit to just one colour

Hat trick

It's not essential to wear a hat at a formal occasion, but if you like hats, a wedding or christening is one of the few places where you can fully indulge yourself without looking like you have been released into community care. When selecting a hat, bear the following in mind:

1

If you are short, avoid wide brims. Don't go wider than your shoulders or you will look like a mushroom.

If you are going to spend a great deal of time outside, be careful about large brims. One gust of wind and you could lose your hat. Make sure you anchor it securely to your hair with a hat pin.

2

Don't forget about your hair. Messy tendrils spilling out of your hat are a no-no. If your hair is long, tie it back.

3

Match your hat to your outfit. If you can't afford a new hat, buy a wide piece of ribbon in a colour that goes with your outfit and cover the band on a plain beige straw.

4

Remember, you can tart up a cheap hat. Feathers and other accessories from a haberdashers can give you a designer look at a fraction of the price.

5

Choose a hat with a deep crown. Shallow crowns look very old-fashioned. Don't choose a hat that looks too small. Bearing in mind the mushroom problem, go for as wide a brim as you can without looking ridiculous. It will look more expensive and modern.

6

Don't even think about a novelty hat. The mother of the bride will not be amused by a baseball cap sprouting a hand clutching a mallet.

And, just in case of disaster

It is wise to take a survival kit with you to a smart do – even if you stay sober, someone else might well decide to pour a glass of red wine down you. A miniature bottle of dry-cleaning fluid and a cloth can be invaluable. Best of all, take a scarf or shawl that tones with your outfit, then if you do manage to tip the soup down yourself and you can't get the stain off with your dry-cleaning fluid, you can drape the scarf over the offending area instead. It's also a good idea to take a spare pair of tights in case you get a ladder.

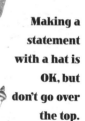

Making a statement with a hat is OK, but don't go over the top.

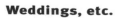

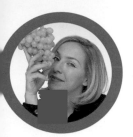

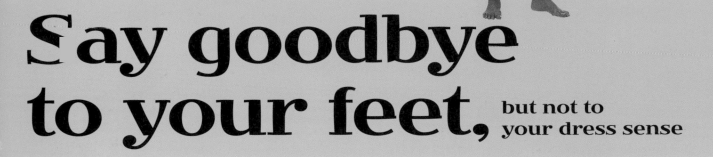

Pregnancy is supposed to be one of the most wonderful experiences a woman can ever go through. So how come she has to go through it wearing some of the most disgusting clothes ever invented?

Say goodbye to your feet, but not to your dress sense

Dresses the size and pattern of especially horrible kitchen curtains, knickers that would be roomy on Jimmy Five Bellies, and as for maternity bras, well they're not exactly seductive, are they?

The assumption is that a pregnant woman is so thrilled to be 'with child' that she'll put on practically anything, so long as it's completely asexual. All those floral prints and frilly collars. What is that about, exactly? Once you're pregnant, it's a bit late to come over all virginal, your bump providing pretty concrete proof that you have actually had sex once in your life at least.

But, it doesn't have to be that way. I met a woman during the last series of *Looking Good* who was eight-and-a-half months pregnant. She was wearing black leather dungarees and she looked fantastic. And she wasn't some designer mum, sitting on a sofa all day being attended to by a battery of New Age therapists. Sarah

had three kids, a husband and a dog. When I met her, she was simultaneously unloading the shopping into the fridge and getting a man to fix her cooker so she could start dinner.

Sarah and women like her are proof that you don't have to transmogrify into some tent-dress-wearing dolt just because you are pregnant. You can look sophisticated, stylish and sexy right up to the birth.

Maternity-wear mistakes

Pregnant women fall into two types. The first group are so delighted to have conceived that they are clearing the racks at Mothercare before they've been pregnant a month. The second group try to ignore their growing stomach and muddle through for as long as they can in normal clothes. Both groups are making a mistake.

You need to acknowledge that your whole shape is changing, not just your waistline. Your bosom will begin to inflate immediately. This can be good news for the AA-cup brigade, not so good news if you start off well endowed. I know one woman whose bra size went up to 38GG! You are also likely to thicken round the hips and, towards the end of the pregnancy, even your back and neck will get bigger, not to forget those swollen ankles.

All these changes need to be accommodated, so don't think you can just sling on a baggy sweater to camouflage them. You'll be able to get away with that in the first few months, but later it will look very peculiar. There is a reason pregnancy knitwear is longer at the front than the back. An ordinary jumper will rise up at the front as it strains to cover your bump.

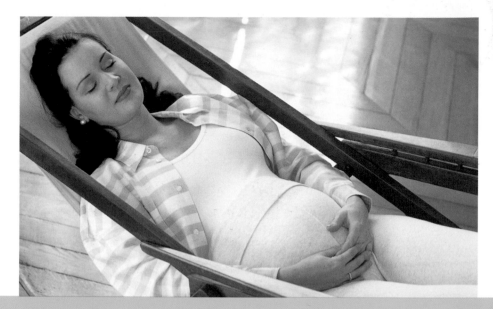

The pre-hippo stage

This is the bit of the pregnancy when you can still struggle into a few of your normal clothes. Its duration depends upon two things:

1 Luck.
2 How much time you spend on the sofa stuffing your face with gherkins and ice cream.

During this time, you may be able to avoid having to buy specific maternity wear. Instead, try the men's department for big tee-shirts or the aforementioned baggy sweaters. Alternatively, just buy from your normal stores a size or two up.

The good thing about elasticated and tie waists is that they can get bigger as you do, but don't go mad on these or baggy tops. It is a fallacy that you should buy things you will want to wear after the pregnancy. Since your post-partum tummy is going to look like a duffle bag for a few weeks, you will be forced to keep wearing

some of your maternity clothing for a while. However, the minute you can get into anything else, you will never want to see that maternity wear again.

Buy more expensive things if they make you feel good. You can always sell the clothes on. Stick an advert up at your antenatal classes so that other mums-to-be can see it. Or just pack the clothes away and hope you have a large family.

The flat shoes are a matter of choice. It will help prevent varicose veins and swollen ankles if you do stick to flats. However, if you are a high heels babe, ration your wear of them. When you're going out, take your high heels in a bag and put them on when you get there. Take them off again as soon as possible afterwards.

'If I think really hard, I can remember what it was like to have a waist.'

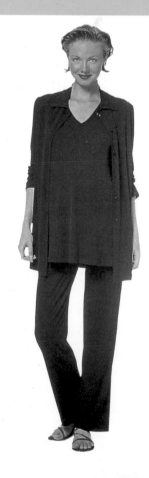

WISE BUYS

loose tee-shirts
big jumpers
tunic tops
skirts and trousers with elasticated waists
jackets with tie waists
flat(ter) shoes

Now you're a hippo

This is the point at which you have trouble getting your knickers on and off. Considering they are of a capaciousness you haven't seen since you were at school and you used to wear 'gym knickers' for sport, it's probably good you can't get too clear a view of how you look in them. Maternity bras are even worse. Not much you can do about either, I'm afraid. Give yourself a squirt with your favourite scent, chant 'I am glamorous, I am glamorous' and remember that pregnancy isn't forever.

It is at the hippo stage that you have to make a choice: do you want to camouflage your bump or flaunt it?

Show it off or cover it up – you choose.

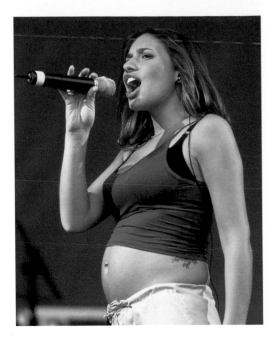

Camouflage

This could be a bit of an uphill struggle. Even if no one noticed your green hue first thing in the morning early on, or the fact that you now have to go to the loo 25 times a day, they are unlikely to have missed your increasing girth.

Still, if you fancy being at least a bit discreet about your pregnancy, then go for more of the tunic tops and baggy tee-shirts over tailored trousers or skirts with elasticated waists. By now, they will have to come from specialist maternity-wear suppliers. The key is to wear tops long enough to cover your tummy and bottom and full enough to give you room to breathe. Don't be tempted to go too big, though. You'll look like a hot-air balloon.

If you feel you're getting really enormous and whale-like, try draping a long scarf around your neck, leaving the ends to dangle to mid-thigh. OK, this might sound a bit pathetic, but it will do something to distract attention away from your midriff. A loose, flowing maxi-length cardigan will also be comfortable and flattering.

If you've got it, flaunt it

This is the All Saints option. At its most extreme, where you actually bare your bulging tummy to the world, it requires enormous bravery, plus an awful lot of olive oil. Flashing stretch marks isn't part of the look.

A less virulent approach is to don a stretchy mini dress that covers and clings to your tummy. This can look brilliant, if you've got the legs to take it. It is really, really unfair, but however proud you are of your baby, you need good legs for the flaunting-it approach. Otherwise you risk just looking Weeble-esque.

Whichever route you decide to take, remember to choose layers of natural fabrics. Pregnancy can be very hot. At least if you're wearing layers you can take things off if you feel yourself overheating.

Pregnancy and the office

Looking professional while you're carting what feels like a sack of potatoes round with you is tricky. For a start, there is a distinct lack of pregnancy office clothing around – does the rag trade think a pregnant woman immediately retires to bake bread at home? What is available is expensive.

Perhaps the best option, at least later in the pregnancy, is to admit defeat on the jacket front and try using tunics over trousers or simple shift dresses instead. To make sure these look smart and business-like, stick to office-type colours – black, navy, beige, grey – and limit yourself to one colour per outfit. Match your tights, shoes, scarf, etc., to your clothing.

If you're on your feet a lot, then you will need to wear flats. Choose simple leather pumps and, if you can, put them on only for important meetings. If you have to walk to and from work, wear trainers and take your smart shoes in a bag.

Pregnancy and posh dos

Evening wear is especially difficult to work round a big tummy. To avoid the galleon-in-full-sail look, steer clear of floaty layers. Keep it as simple and fitted as you can. Go tight over the bits of you that are still slim –

shoulders, arms, legs – and looser where you have expanded. Again, if you have good legs, you've got a head start.

One thing that all pregnant women, whether they have legs like tree trunks or saplings, can really show off is their cleavages. It is likely to be spectacular, so make the most of it. Empire line frocks, which are draped from a fitted bodice, are wonderful on pregnant women.

I've had the baby, so why do I still feel fat?

I remember reading a hideous story about actress Jane Seymour. When she had given birth to her twins she weighed less than she had before she was pregnant. She weighed LESS! Most women aren't so lucky. You're going to be carrying around a spare tyre for a minimum of a few weeks yet, so resist the temptation to burn your maternity clothing.

Instead, cheat a little. If you haven't already got bodyshaper tights, go and buy some. Forget whose child you've just had; when you've tried bodyshapers, you'll want to have their inventor's child. If you really want to do battle with the tum, wear control knickers as well.

As far as clothes are concerned, think of it as a fat day that's just going on a bit. Look at the 'Fat Days' chapter on page 22. Most of the tips there are as good for hiding post-pregnancy flub. The most important thing, though, is to enjoy your pregnancy. This is one time when it's OK to let things slide a little and waddle about like an overfed penguin. It's not your fault. You're pregnant.

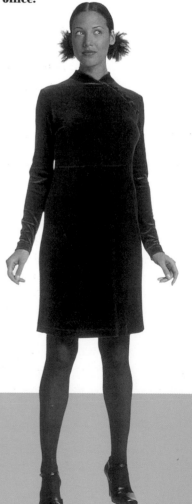

Not a Peter Pan collar in sight. Smart maternity wear for the office.

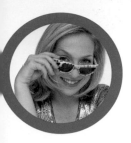

I love watching holiday programmes on TV. What I don't like so much is when the camera leaves the scenery and zooms in on people. Invariably these people are young, female and there isn't an inch of cellulite in sight.

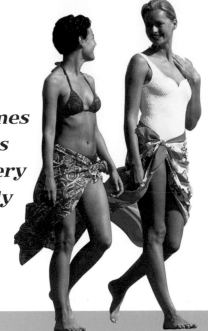

No, you can't wear your sarong in the sea

Confronted with perfect bodies, I suddenly go right off a resort.

Forget exchange rates, average rainfall or flight time, I think holiday programmes should include an estimate of the likely dress size of everyone at a particular destination as a matter of urgency. If the beach I'm going to will be stuffed with skinny girls, then I'm going to have to spend my entire holiday holding my tummy in. And what kind of holiday is that? Judith Chalmers, show me a place where everyone is size 26 and over and I'll be on the next plane.

I know I'm not alone. Shop changing-room queues in July are full of women with gritted teeth, clutching bikinis and bracing themselves for the sight of their spare tyres in artificial light. Then, as that

Old-fashioned swimsuits – at least you got to cover up a little.

little strip of plastic scratches in all the wrong places, you try to fold excess flesh into tiny knickers and fail. Frankly, it's depressing, isn't it?

The first rule of swimwear buying – get it over with early

The mistake most of us make is to leave buying a swimsuit until the last minute. This usually means some time at the end of July, precisely the point at which all stock, including swimwear, is at its lowest. The only swimwear left in July is the really odd stuff, or things that would only fit Barbie.

There are usually two reasons why you didn't get round to buying it before:

1

You assume you can get into last year's swimsuit, without realizing that last year's model is in fact a decade old, no longer fits you anywhere and has a cigarette burn under one armpit.

2

You are on a diet and you don't want to try a swimsuit on until you reach your target weight. The problem is you've been on that diet since January, it's now July and you've actually put on half a stone.

If you can, try to buy your swimsuit early. You will have so much more choice and you won't have to resort to panic buying.

I remember one year buying a bikini the day before my take-off. The shop didn't have my size, so I ended up buying one that needed a foot taken out of the back. That night I went for a pre-holiday drink, meaning to alter my cossie when I got home. It wasn't until I was on my holiday and went to put on my bikini that I realized I had been so sozzled I'd used a darning needle and the wrong-coloured thread.

One piece or two?

Most women assume that a one-piece swimsuit will automatically be more flattering, simply because it covers more. However, if you have a long body and short legs, a bikini can look much better. One-piece swimsuits accentuate the length of your body, while two shorten it.

I'll have a costume in any colour so long as it's black

There is no doubt that black is the most slimming colour for a swimsuit. So, if you want to play safe, by all means buy black. However, you should bear in mind that black is not kind to pale skin. So while it

might reduce your bottom, your new black costume could also make you look alarmingly consumptive.

It's a good idea, therefore, to take two swimsuits on holiday with you – one in a pastel colour and one black. The pastel one you wear the first week of your holiday, while you are still working on your tan. Then, when you have achieved a golden glow, you swap to the black one. An added benefit of doing a swapsy is that you've probably been stuffing yourself solidly for seven days, so by the second week of a fortnight away you'll need the slimming properties of black.

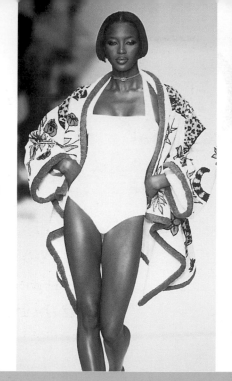

Hallelujah for the beach wrap (not that Naomi needs one).

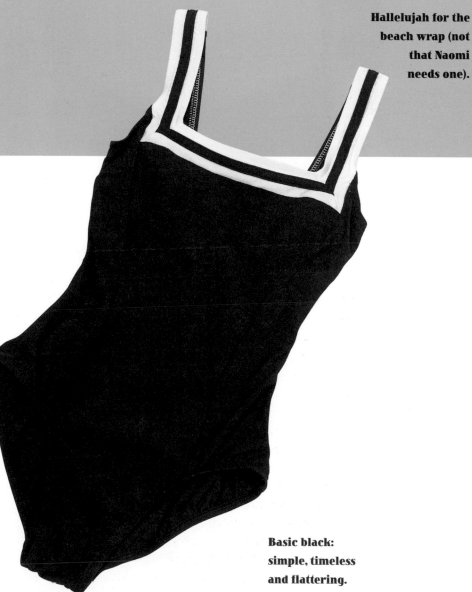

Basic black: simple, timeless and flattering.

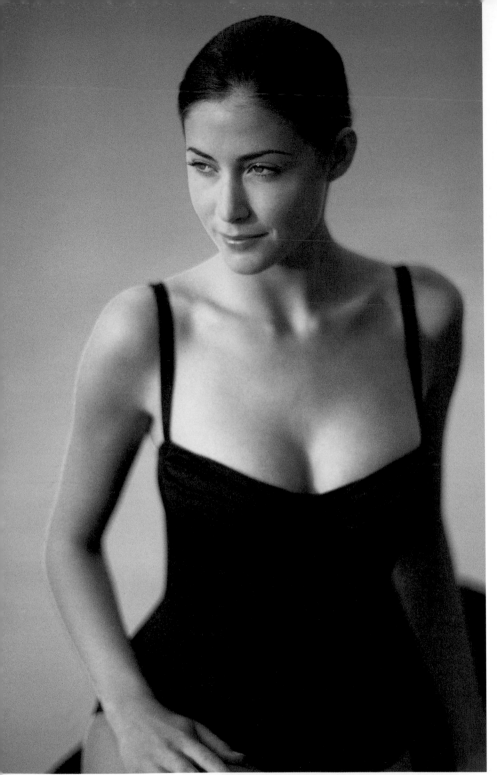

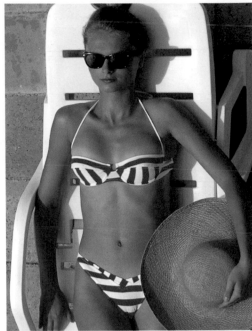

bigger bottoms and thighs), hourglasses (who have large busts and hips, and small waists) and ironing boards (who go straight up and down).

If you're an apple shape

A one-piece will definitely be best on you. You need to slim the middle section. Use vertical stripes or panels to whittle your waist. Avoid halter necks and high legs. You want the impression of width at the top and bottom of the suit to make the waist look narrower. A skirted bottom half and wide-set shoulder straps will be most flattering.

If you're a pear shape

It's your bottom half that you need to slim down. So whether you're going for a one- or two-piece, make sure the bottom half is black. High-cut legs will be a disaster on you, but so will longer '40s-style big knickers. A compromise between the two, with perhaps a little matching skating skirt you could tie over the top, would be ideal.

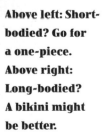

Above left: Short-bodied? Go for a one-piece. Above right: Long-bodied? A bikini might be better.

How to choose the right swimsuit for your shape

First, take a long hard look at yourself in a full-length mirror at home. You need to work out what body shape you have. For convenience we will divide everyone into apples (who collect weight round the middle), pears (who have small busts and

SWIMWEAR NO-NOS

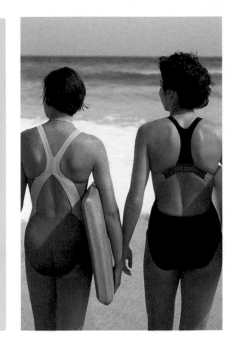

There are some swimwear ideas that don't suit anybody:

1 ANYTHING IN WHITE, UNLESS IT'S WELL-LINED — BOUND TO GO SEE-THROUGH IN WATER **2** ANYTHING IN SALMON PINK — GET SUNBURN AND YOU'LL LOOK EXACTLY LIKE A LOBSTER **3** ONE-PIECES WITH HOLES OR LACING UP THE SIDES — EVEN IF YOUR FLESH DOESN'T BULGE OUT OF THE GAPS, YOU'LL GET A VERY STRANGE TAN **4** ANYTHING WITH METAL BUCKLES OR BUTTONS ON — THEY WILL DIG INTO YOU WHEN YOU LIE DOWN AND IF YOU SIT UP, THEY'LL GET HOT ENOUGH TO GIVE YOU A THIRD-DEGREE BURN

To balance a heavier bottom half, try a lighter colour on top. Also, if you have a small bust, tie-fronted designs, or those with ruching, gathering and frills across the cleavage, will give the impression of a fuller bosom.

If you're an hour-glass shape

Your small waist may be your most prized feature, but if you draw attention to it, you risk making your bust and hips look enormous. A two-piece suit might be best on you. Use a dark colour to slim top and bottom.

For a heavy bust, bra-style bikini tops are usually best. You definitely need support, so look out for underwiring or preformed cups. Do not even think about a bandeau style — lean forward on your sun-lounger and the top will fold over and expose you to the world.

If you're an ironing-board shape

The good news is you don't have to worry too much about support. Sporty, racer-back designs and string-sided bikinis will look good on you.

If you're concerned about a small bust, choose padded or underwired cups to push up what you have. Then add draping or ruching to improve the impression of curves. Halter necks also push bosoms together, making them look bigger.

Sporty shapes are fine on the super-skinny. Otherwise it's on with a sarong (below).

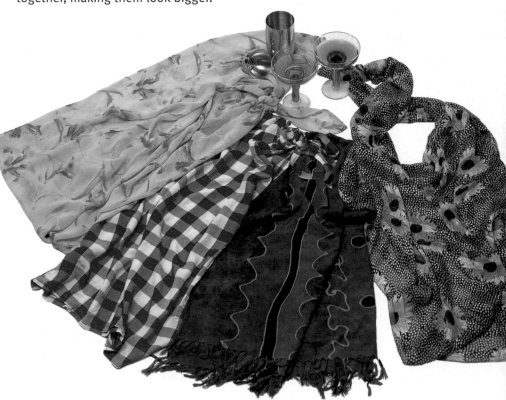

Thank goodness for the sarong

The sarong has to be one of the best fashion inventions ever. In the old days (well, my childhood anyway) the only ways to cover your bottom when you went to get an ice-cream were to tie a towel round yourself or to put on one of those towelling capes you used to change underneath.

These days you can conceal all the wobbly bits and be stylish too.

Still, if the idea of the sarong is pure brilliance, actually tying one is quite difficult. First off, when you buy a sarong, select one with a width no larger than the length between your waist and ankle. The length should be enough to go around you one-and-a-half times.

Not all men are Adonises on the beach, either

Do men worry how they look in their swimming trunks? On the whole, no. This is both a blessing – for them – and a curse – for the rest of us. How many times have you seen a guy with the most enormous beer belly in a posing pouch and gone right off your rum cocktail?

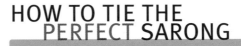

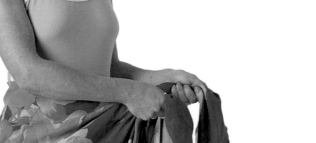

Don't tie yourself in knots. Here's the right way to tie a sarong.

HOW TO TIE THE PERFECT SARONG

1

Take the fabric and pass it behind you so that the long sides are parallel with the ground (just as you would if you were about to towel-dry your bottom).

2

Put the ends together and pull the sarong round you so that both ends are on your left.

3

Twist the ends separately so that the fabric begins to drape.

4

Knot the ends on the left of your waist with a reef knot.

It's the twisting that gives your sarong the right draped look. You can also make the sarong into a dress if you want to cover more of yourself.

86

HOW TO TIE THE PERFECT SARONG DRESS

1

With the long sides parallel with the ground, pass the sarong behind you and lift it up until it is armpit level.

2

Put the two ends together in front of you.

3

Twist the ends separately until the fabric drapes.

4

Take the twisted ends and twist them round each other a couple of times.

5

Pass the twisted ends round your neck and knot at the back.

There are other cover-up options around. Moroccan-style linen jellabahs and towelling bath robes in white are cool and comfortable.

For younger men in their teens and twenties, '6os-style hipster trunks are now back in. However, once a man can no longer balance a pint of lager on his tummy, presumably because he's poured too many down his neck, he should be pleaded with to avoid stretchy swimwear. Baggy swimming shorts, as long as they are in a plain colour, are much more seemly. And if he insists on wearing his favourite trunks, despite the fact they're horrible? Offer to do his packing for him, then just forget to pack them.

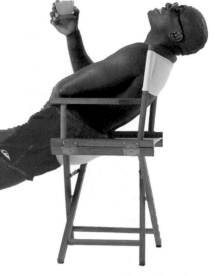

Swim shorts – the most flattering choice for most men.

THE THREE SWIMWEAR STYLES NO MAN SHOULD EVER WEAR

1 TINY SPEEDOS **2** G-STRING SPEEDOS

3 LURID SURF SHORTS

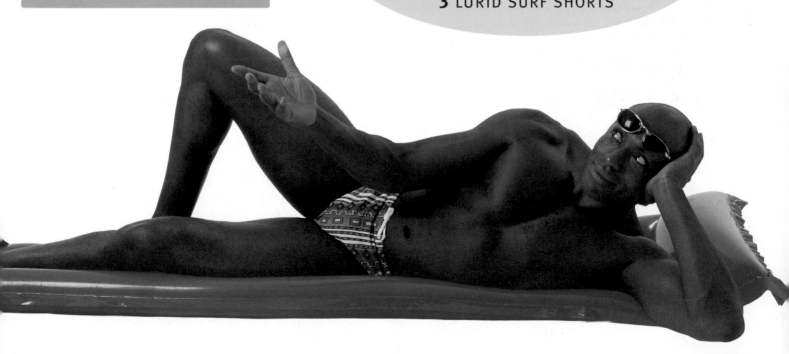

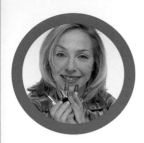

There is something miraculous about make-up. You can get up in the morning with the most stonking hang-over, a fresh spot and eye bags the size of holdalls and 20 minutes later emerge looking, well, if not quite like a Miss World, certainly a thousand times better than you did first thing.

Is this really the best I'm going to look all day?

Not only capable of giving an enormous physical lift, cosmetics are also marvellous psychologically. Got an important meeting? Stick some lipstick on, love. Got a broken heart? Try a bit more blusher, honey, you'll feel a whole lot better. Never mind aspirin – the best medicine for almost any female condition is a quick delve in the old make-up bag. They don't call it warpaint for nothing, you know.

That's the way it should be. The problem is no one teaches you how to put make-up on properly. When I was a teenager, about the only information on the correct application of make-up came in little diagrams in *Jackie* magazine. They didn't look like anyone I knew and always featured at least four colours of eyeshadow. I could only run to a grey kohl pencil and a tester rouge from Rimmel.

These days things are both better and worse. Better because there is more information around. Worse because there is so much more make-up available. Things have got complicated. Go into a branch of Boots now and there are at least 20 make-up stands. All are crammed with powders and pencils, gels, creams and polishes. They look like old-fashioned Woolworth's Pick-and-Mix counters. Except, pick the wrong product and that mistake is considerably more expensive than buying a humbug instead of a chocolate eclair.

Cosmetics graveyard

Every woman has one of these. It is filled with old make-up that she bought and either never wore or wore once and decided she looked dreadful in it, so never wore it again. If you added up the prices on all the stuff in your cosmetics graveyard it would probably come to hundreds of pounds.

You have only one choice: bin the lot. It might stick in your throat to throw away all this stuff, but make-up doesn't last indefinitely. Just like food, it goes off. Mascaras and eye pencils are among the most dangerous things to hold on to. They harbour bacteria. If you dig them out and use them when they've been lying fallow for a year, you could give yourself an eye infection. And it's no use saying your Auntie Maude has had the same block mascara for 20 years; she's lucky if she can still see out of both eyes.

Chill out

Make-up is not designed to last more than six months; in the case of mascara, three months. That's how often you should change it, even if it's not finished. One way to make make-up last longer is to put it in the fridge. This will stop it going off and double the time it lasts.

Of course, this could be a bit inconvenient. You try finding your mascara first thing in the morning, when you're bleary eyed and it's rolled behind a Mr Man yoghurt and fallen down the back of the fridge. Good luck.

How to slay yourself a make-up dragon

Behind every cosmetics counter is a make-up dragon. She's the one wearing an inch of foundation. It's a mystery why they do this. I for one take a look at those girls and it puts me right off buying from them lest I end up looking as terrifyingly over made-up.

One way to slay a make-up dragon is to buy make-up from those cheaper brands that don't employ demonstrators. Rimmel, Bourjois and L'Oréal (among others) allow you to browse without coming under the evil eye of a member of staff.

But perhaps you'd like some advice? Well, then you're going to have to deal with the harridan behind the counter. Take a deep breath and ask your question, but remember she is there to sell you things. These companies might sell beauty as a science, but it's doubtful that your make-up dragon has a PhD in AHAs – a GCSE in home economics, more like. Don't be intimidated.

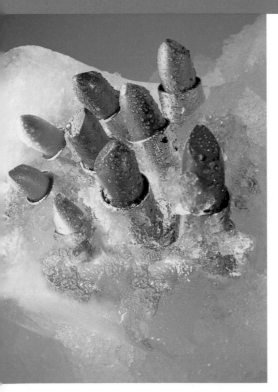

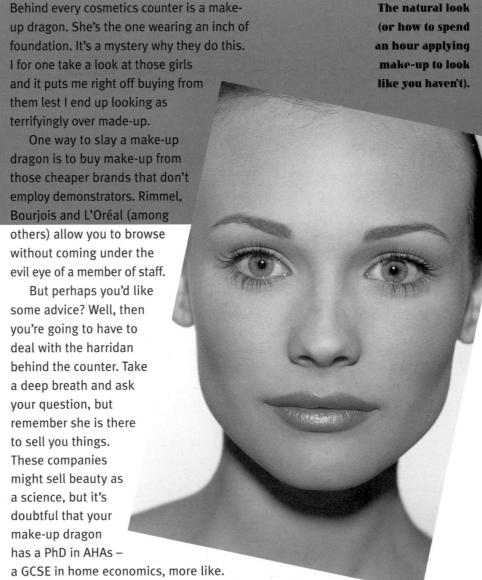

The natural look (or how to spend an hour applying make-up to look like you haven't).

Make-over and out?

One useful service that the make-up dragons do offer is a free make-over. You usually have to book these in advance by either calling the counter on the phone or going in and asking a member of staff. You are not forced to buy the products they use afterwards, although you might find you come under a certain amount of pressure to do so.

The quality of the make-up on offer varies enormously. So before you book your make-over, take a walk around a cosmetics hall. Bear in mind that the sort of make-up look you will be given is likely to be similar to that displayed on the various make-up dragons. Choose the counter with someone behind it who has the sort of style you are looking for.

The era when there was little choice – it was satsuma face or nothing – is over, happily. If you want classic glamour, book a make-over at one of the well-established names such as Yves Saint Laurent, Chanel, Clinique, or Estée Lauder. If you want a younger, trendier look, try Mac, Bobby Brown or François Nars. At the very least you'll be pampered for 15 minutes for free. At the worst, you'll look ridiculous and have to nip to the nearest ladies and wash it all off again.

Way too weird – some looks are best left to the catwalk.

Nailing a beauty myth

The beauty industry is predicated on the myth that you can buy beauty out of a bottle and that the more you spend, the more beautiful you will look. On a rational level, no sensible woman believes this. But deep down we secretly want to believe it. We need to believe it. If we can buy a wrinkle-free complexion, sparkly eyes and high cheekbones over the counter, then we don't

have to give up smiling and drinking, or go to the gym.

Make-up might be magic, but it can't do miracles. It is basically just pots of different coloured gunge that either does or doesn't look pretty on the face. Whether you pay a huge amount for this gunge or just a few pounds, the difference is subjective. That is not to say there aren't differences between cheap and expensive brands.

There are several:

1 Expensive brands are packaged better.
2 Expensive brands often have a high pigment content, meaning you need to use less of them and they last longer.
3 Expensive brands usually have the most up-to-date colours.

The packaging issue is a matter of personal taste. Yes, there is something enormously satisfying about snapping shut a Chanel powder compact. It feels terribly glamorous to apply Yves Saint Laurent eyeshadow. If your life is enhanced by having a matching set of mirrored Clinique eyeshadow boxes, then go ahead. But it's not essential.

As for the pigment question, put a designer eyeshadow next to a value brand and the likelihood is that it will take less of the former to get a good, deep colour. This means that it might work out cheaper in the long run to buy the more expensive one.

However, that supposes that you won't go off the eyeshadow after a few months. Most of us have got drawers full of colours we no longer like. So, if it's a colour you've been using for years and you know you'll keep using it, then maybe buy the designer version; if not, stick to cheap brands.

It is absolutely true that if you want really fashionable colours, you have to buy the expensive brands. Chanel's Rouge Noir nail polish is a case in point. It was at least nine months before the other labels caught up and produced a deep, dark red that could compete with Rouge Noir.

However, in the same way that high-street fashion chains have speeded up, so the gap between designer make-up lines and cheaper ones is narrowing. If you want really trendy colours take a look at Rimmel, Boots 17 and L'Oréal.

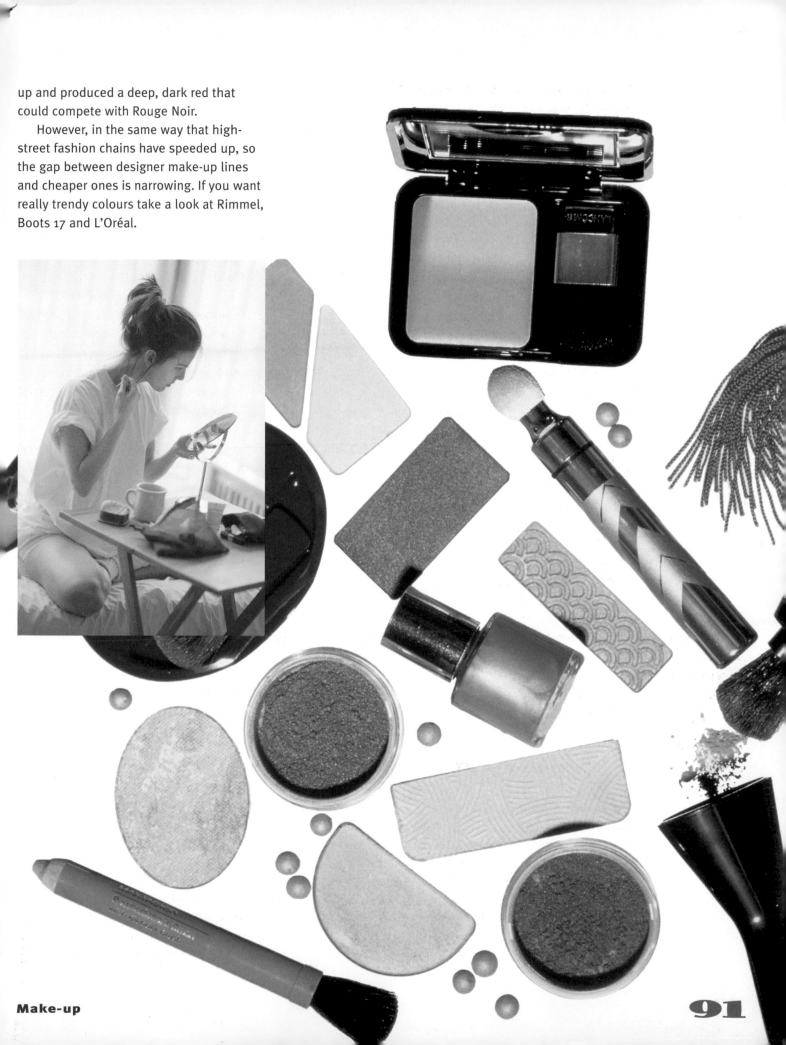

English rose v olive skin

Before you buy any make-up you need to establish your skin colour. This might seem obvious. You are either pale, tanned, Asian or black, right? Wrong. It is the hue not the depth of colour that is important. People's skins fall into two types. They are either pink or yellow toned. And you might think that because you are pale, you are pink. Think again. Most of us have a yellow tone to our skin, no matter how pallid we look. Most black and Asian skins are yellow toned.

If you are one of those who is not obviously either pink or yellow toned, then the easiest way to work out which you are is to hold the inside of your arm next to a definite yellow or pink. Older women are almost invariably pink toned, Asian women almost always yellow. I'm not suggesting you accost someone in the street, but find a member of your family or a friend, go into the daylight and compare arms.

Once you have worked that out, it should be a guide to buying the correct shade of foundation, which are also pink or yellow toned. Ask the assistant which one has the tone you want, put some on your face – don't bother with your arm, it never works – and go out into the daylight with a mirror to see how it looks. Keep doing this until you find the perfect match. Yes, you might look stupid, but it's the only way to get the perfect match. And remember, that is what you are looking for – a PERFECT match with your skin tone.

The tone of your skin also determines what eyeshadows, lipsticks and blushers

Colour me beautiful – test out make-up before you buy.

you should wear. Choose carefully and you won't end up looking like a clown.

If you have a pink-toned skin

Look for cool, blue-ish make-up. Pink lipsticks, rather than reds and browns. Grey, blue and lilac eyeshadows, rather than peaches and tawny shades. All will have an affinity with your skin.

If you have a yellow-toned skin

Your skin needs warm colours to look ' healthy. Brown and gold eyeshadows will look good, as will warm reddish lipsticks. You can go for a fuchsia lip colour if you like. It will not look in the least bit natural, but it will look very striking.

Now you're ready to go shopping. So what do you buy?

There is no reason for you to buy acres of stuff. The best make-up bags are neat and organized. Indeed, you can double up on products to save space and money. A blusher can be used as an eyeshadow. An eyeshadow can double as an eyebrow colour. Experiment.

YOUR MAKE-UP ESSENTIALS

If you want to start from scratch, this is what your make-up bag should contain:

foundation

concealer

loose translucent powder

mascara

blusher

eyeshadow

lip pencil

lipstick

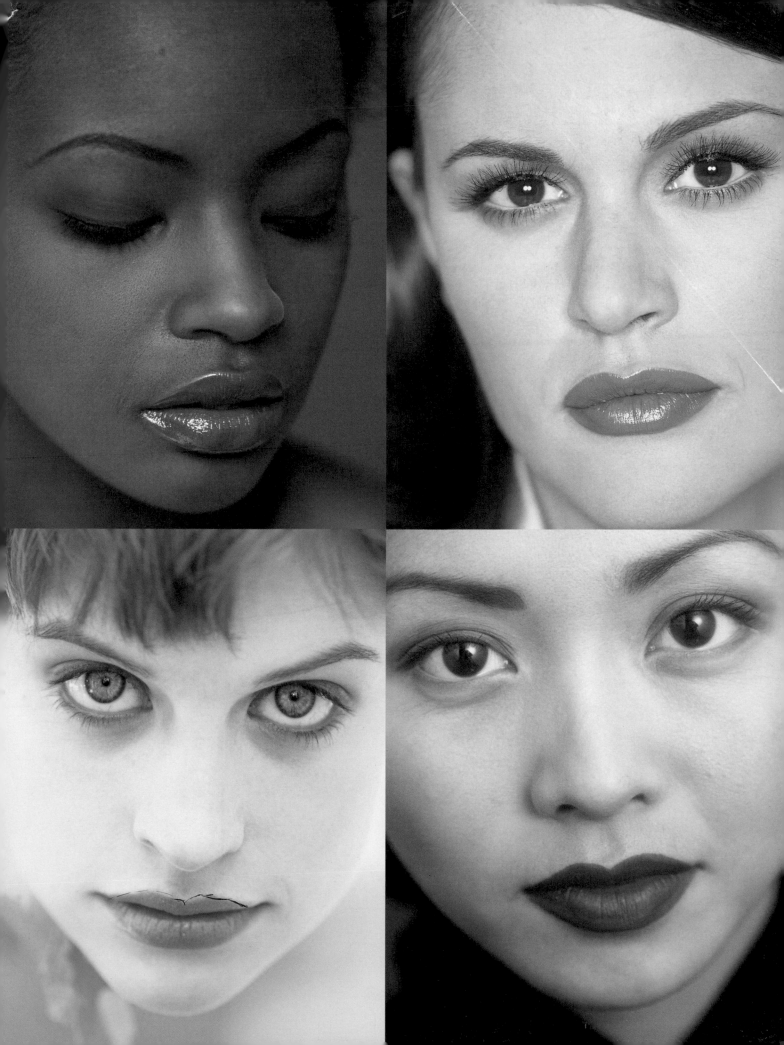

Pencil, powder or cream?

This is a matter of taste. I find creams very difficult to handle. When I'm using a cream eyeshadow, I get more under my fingernails than I ever do on my eyelid. Cream blushers can also be difficult to blend.

Still, two things that I think are best as a cream or liquid are foundation and concealer. Powder foundations go on very quickly. They offer instant coverage. But at a price. They aren't very moisturizing and can collect in your wrinkles. You can end up looking more raddled than when you started. Powder eyeshadows on an older woman have the same effect.

Pencils also have their downside. Eye pencils can drag the eye, especially if you have older skin. But they are very good at delivering long-lasting colour. If you're going out for the evening and will be doing a lot of eating and drinking, ditch the lipstick. Use a lip pencil all over your lips instead. It will last much longer.

My preference is for powder as an eyeshadow and as an eyebrow colour. It is easy to apply and blend as an eyeshadow and, if you add a couple of drops of water and use a fine eyeliner brush, also works incredibly well as an eyeliner. If you have blonde, red, or any unusual colour of hair, finding an eyebrow pencil that matches exactly is difficult. With powder you can mix your own exact shade.

Good brushes are essential. You can rely on those little sponge applicators you get

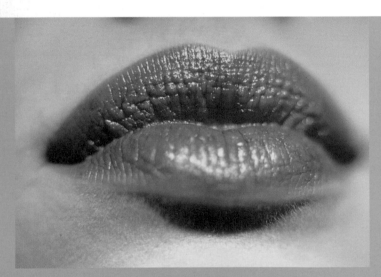

The perfect lips – or why you really should use a lip brush.

MAKE-UP TOOLS YOU REALLY NEED

eyeshadow brush

angled eyebrow brush

fine eyeliner brush

blusher brush

large powder brush

lipbrush

powder puff

eyebrow tweezers

AND SOME YOU DON'T

1 FOAM WEDGES
Ever wondered what those little wedges of foam you see in packets are for? So make-up manufacturers can get you to use loads of foundation and waste most of it. Don't buy them.

2 EYELASH CURLERS
Expensive torture instruments. If you don't clean them regularly you will pull out all your eyelashes.

3 CLEAR MASCARA
Supposedly useful for arranging naturally long eyelashes. Who has those? Some also use it to tame wild eyebrows, but we're getting a bit Princess and the pea here, aren't we? Waste of time.

4 LIPSTICK SEALER
This is the clear stuff you paint on to your lips to prevent your lipstick running. It works, yes, but your lips set like concrete.

free with most eyeshadows, but did Michelangelo paint the Sistine Chapel with one of those? I think not. You will get a better result if you use a brush. That said, brushes are expensive. It is a false economy to buy them in a set. You will end up only ever using a couple of them and the rest will be useless. Buy your brushes singly.

Get yourself a powder puff, by which I mean one of those fabric-covered round sponges. This is for pressing powder into your face. It should be washable. Tweezers are essential because if you're going to go to all the trouble of putting your eyeshadow on with brushes, you want a good frame for your eyes. No pain, no gain.

You've now got your kit. Here's what to do with it.

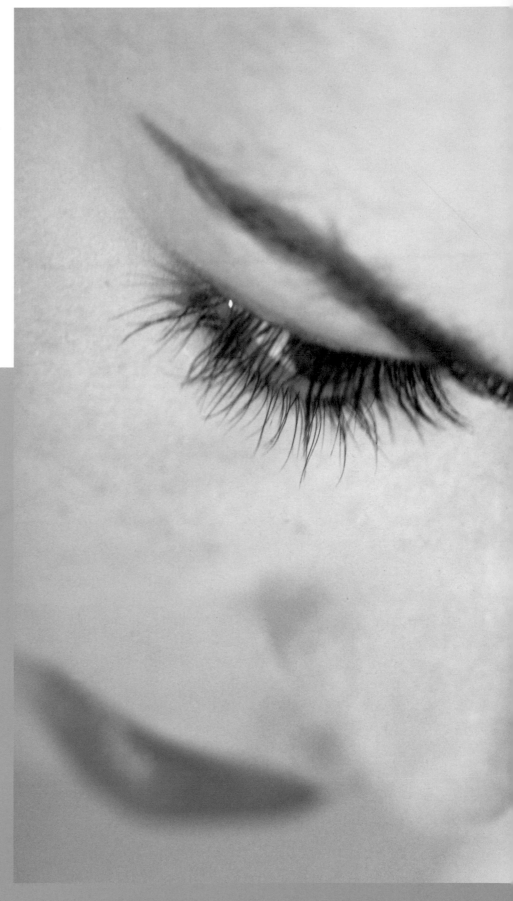

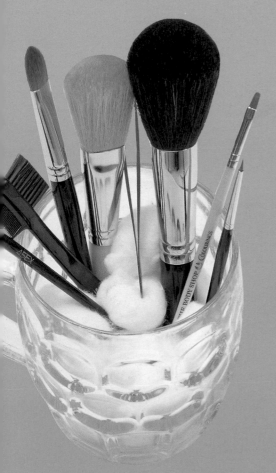

STEP-BY-STEP GUIDE TO A
BASIC MAKE-UP

1   Start with a clean face, then, using your fingers, apply the foundation. Don't put too much on – it will make you look older. Foundation is for evening out your tone, not obliterating every last blemish. Blend, blend, blend.

2   Concealer. This is where you deal with serious problems – spots, broken veins, blotchiness. Use your fingers to dab it on.

3   Take a soft powder puff and press translucent powder all over your face, except under your eyes, where it is better to use a brush. Use this brush again all over your face to remove excess powder.

A trick that make-up artists use is to add a little extra powder underneath your eye, so that if eyeshadow falls down while you are applying it, you can simply brush it off.

4   Use a neutral colour of eyeshadow as a base – beigy if you've yellow skin, pinky if you haven't. Use your eyeshadow brush to put it all over your lids and brow bone, up to the brows.

5   Take a slightly darker colour and put this in your eye sockets. Blend well.

6   Take your eyeliner brush and use it to add a couple of drops of water to either a black or a dark brown eyeshadow. Blend and draw a line close to the lashes on your upper eyelid. Wing up slightly on the outside corner. Apply another line along the bottom set of lashes. Leave to dry, then soften the line with your eyeshadow brush.

7   Use your eyebrow brush and a colour close to your natural eyebrow shade to emphasize the shape of your brows and fill in any gaps. You will have already used the tweezers to pluck out any strays.

8   Apply mascara using a windscreen wiper motion to top and bottom lashes. This makes sure you get it on both sides of the lashes, enabling you to build them better. Two thin coats is better than one heavy coat.

9   Using your blusher brush, select a blusher colour close to your own natural blush and apply powder to the apples of your cheeks. A good tip is to smile so that you can see where your apples are. Blend up towards your temples, but steer clear of the Mars Bar effect.

10   Take a lip pencil and outline your lips. Then fill in with lipstick using your lip brush. It's really important to have a matching lip pencil and lipstick. A dark lip line is harsh and very ageing. If you can't afford a set of lip liners, just go with the lipstick on its own. Blot lips, or use a lip gloss.

A FEW
TRADE SECRETS

HOW TO MAKE YOUR EYES LOOK INSTANTLY BRIGHTER

Apply a small amount of white eye-shadow to the corners of your eyes nearest to your nose.

HOW TO MAKE YOUR EYES LOOK BIGGER

Pluck your eyebrows. Leave the half of the eyebrow nearest your nose more or less unscathed. Pluck above your nose if you need to. However, concentrate on the ends. Thin them out, plucking from the bottom only. This will give you an instant eye lift.

HOW TO GIVE YOURSELF CHEEKBONES IF YOU HAVEN'T GOT ANY

Use a slightly iridescent highlighter powder in the gap below your eye and above your blusher. Blend this into your blusher. Then, under your blusher, use a slightly browner powder to hollow out your cheeks. Go easy, though, or you could end up looking like a drag queen. This definitely works best in dim light.

HOW TO MAKE YOUR LIPS LOOK FULLER

Use two colours of lipstick at once. The darker colour goes on the outside edges of you lips. The lighter shade fills in the middle.

HOW TO MAKE YOUR LIPSTICK LAST LONGER

Apply a layer of foundation and powder to your lips before you put your lipstick on. This will give the lipstick something to grip to and will help it stay on. Another tip is to lick the rim of a glass before you drink from it. Your lipstick won't come off on it.

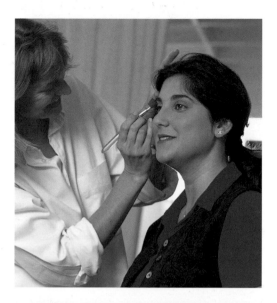

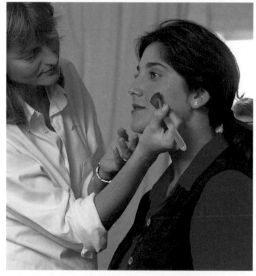

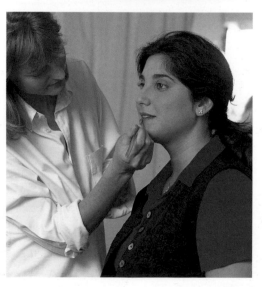

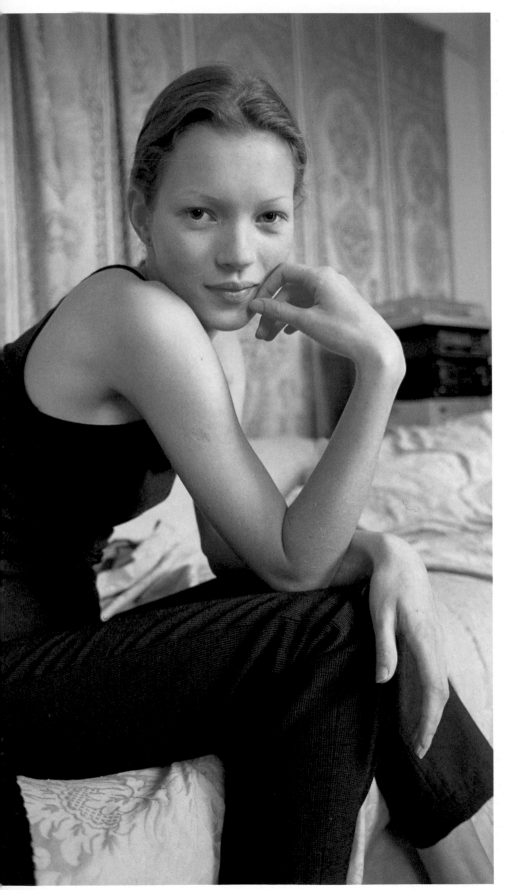

So what happened to the natural look?

The idea of the natural look is a good one. You enhance the features you already have to acquire a fabulous healthy glow. But what if those natural features aren't so wonderful? The great thing about make-up for most of us is that it changes the way we look. We start off looking grotty and end up looking gorgeous. If you are a supermodel (like Kate Moss, left) then the natural look works just perfectly. If, like the rest of us, you need some help, forget it.

That's not to say you have to spend four hours every morning applying a mask. The women who do that are sad. There is a way to make yourself look better fast.

QUICK FIXES

However much care you have taken over your make-up in the morning, by evening it's going to need a repair job. There are good and bad ways of doing this.

DON'T apply more foundation over the top of old foundation. That's slutsville. Besides, it will look like you're wearing rice pudding.

DON'T apply more mascara over old mascara. It will look like lumpy rice pudding.

DO remove foundation from the bits of your face that have seen the worst wear and tear – your nose, around your mouth and under your eyes probably – and reapply.

DO put an iridescent eyeshadow over the top of any existing ones to add a bit of sparkle.

DO reapply your lipstick and add some gloss.

A lick and a promise

Most of us haven't got the time to use all the tricks of the trade every day. We have five minutes before we've got to be out the door. If that's the case, you can pare down your make-up to just a quick once over with a translucent powder compact, some mascara, blusher and a tinted lip gloss. The transformation won't be so dramatic but hey, it's better than nothing.

Yes, you do have to take it off at night

The worst thing about make-up is the taking off bit. But if you don't take it off, two things will happen:

1 You will get spots. Your skin needs to be able to breathe and if it's clogged with foundation it will break out.
2 Your pillows will get nasty brown streaks and black smudges on them.

It's tempting after a hard night on the tiles to just fall (or pass out) into bed. Once in a blue moon this won't do you any harm. But as a rule, be firm with yourself. Cleanse, tone and moisturize, girls.

But what if I get lucky?

Knowing at what point in a relationship he is ready to see you au naturel is tricky. You don't want to scare him off by letting him see you completely bare faced on the second date, but the vision of you first thing in the morning with last night's make-up congealed on your face is also pretty scary.

I know girls who have got out of bed at six a.m. the morning after the night before to reapply a full face of make-up. The thing is, he's so knackered from the night before, he doesn't notice anyway. You're not on *Dallas*. He won't switch on the light at three in the morning and expect you to be looking radiant.

A gradual approach is probably best. Start by wiping off your lipstick. Then remove the foundation and eyeshadow. Leave the mascara and perhaps a bit of blusher till last. Only when you're sure he won't run screaming from the room do you start rubbing in the cold cream before bed.

If you're really concerned about being seen without make-up, only date men who are short sighted. Once he's taken off his contact lenses, you will be in a beautiful haze however little make-up you're wearing.

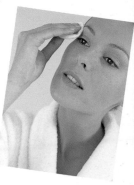

What goes on must come off – unless you want to look like a panda in the morning.

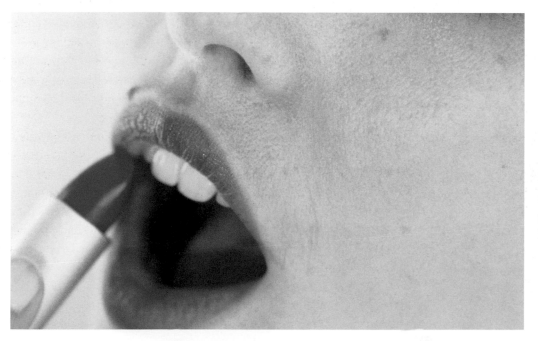

A fresh coat of glossy lipstick gives an instant lift to your looks.

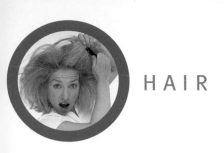

HAIR

When it comes to traumatic events, a visit to the hairdresser has to be up there with trips to the dentist and the gynaecologist.

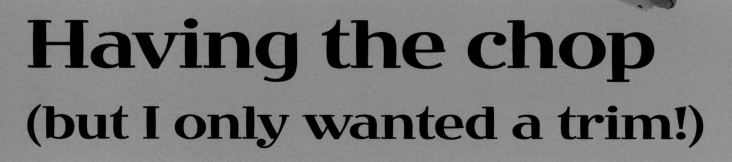

Having the chop
(but I only wanted a trim!)

After visits to the dentist or gynaecologist you walk out looking, on the outside anyway, roughly the same. With the hairdresser there is a very real possibility that you will walk out looking horrendous. And it's no use saying, 'Oh well, it'll grow back,' because it takes months to do that.

I remember girls at school crying for days over bad perms. If anyone else said 'Don't worry. The curls will loosen up', they just wailed all the louder. There was one occasion when my sister had a hair disaster. She went off to get her hair dyed platinum and cut into a short crop. When she arrived home she looked like a light bulb. They had cut her hair one length all over and dyed it yellow. She took one look at my appalled face and burst into tears.

But we can't put all the blame on hairdressers. Yes, there are some bad ones,

One girl, a million copycat haircuts. Jennifer Aniston models 'The Rachel'.

especially if they are inexperienced. If you spend £2.50 to have your hair cut on a student night, you are pretty much dicing with death. That person with the scissors might well never have held a pair before. If you come out looking even halfway decent, you are very lucky indeed.

Hairdressers do their best to give us the look we want. It is in their interests to please us. We might come back and spend more money. Plus, they have to listen to us witter on about our holidays, our boyfriends, what we gave the cat last night for dinner. It's a wonder more murders aren't committed in the crimper's chair. We, the customers, must be so boring. When there is a falling out, it's usually because either we haven't made ourselves understood, or we have asked them to do the impossible.

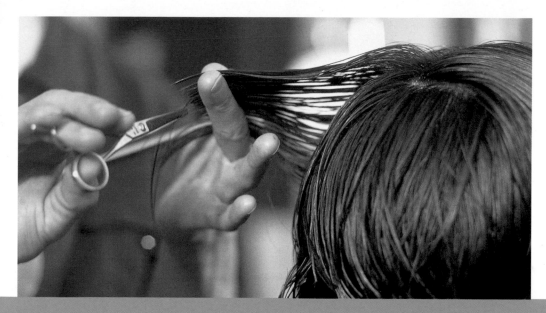

I said I wanted a Demi Moore, not a Roger Moore!

The first rule of hairdressing is that the customer and the hairdresser must understand each other. So, if you really do want only a trim, make sure you say so, and get confirmation that you have been understood. Ask your hairdresser how much he or she is going to cut off and get them to show you. Then, if it is too much, say so.

If you are contemplating a more radical style, look through magazines and find something that looks the way you want your hair to look. Far from being insulted by this, most hairdressers welcome some firm idea of what you want. If you are really nervous about going for a change, then book in for a consultation separate from your haircut. The hairdresser might charge you for this – after all, it could take 20 minutes of his or her time – but you can discuss ideas and go away to think about it before actually having the chop.

Hairdresser speak

Having said that you must make yourself clear, what complicates this is that hairdressers often use a strange language. Only distantly related to English, it is two parts flattery to one part subtle sarcasm. So you know what he or she is really saying, here's a quick guide:

Hairdresser says: 'Perhaps it's time to freshen up your colour.'
Hairdresser means: 'When did you last have your roots done? They are terrible.'

Hairdresser says: 'I'm just going to blunt off the ends.'
Hairdresser means: 'You've got so many split ends, I'm going to have to cut a foot off the back just to get it level.'

Hairdresser says: 'Have you considered growing out your fringe? A more swept-back style would really bring out your cheekbones.'
Hairdresser means: 'That fringe makes your face look like a potato. For God's sake get rid of it.'

Asking for the impossible

Taking along a picture from a magazine is all very well, but if you have a dark brown crop and you produce a snap of Claudia Schiffer, you are being a bit hopeful, aren't you? You're seeing a hairdresser not a plastic surgeon.

'Oops, you did say you wanted a Sinead O'Connor, didn't you?'

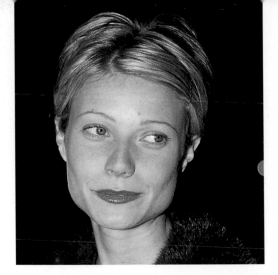

To fringe or not to fringe? Study your face before getting the chop or go for a Gwyneth Paltrow compromise.

BEFORE YOU CHOOSE YOUR NEW STYLE, YOU NEED TO CONSIDER THREE THINGS:

1

FACE SHAPE

Your face shape dictates what style will flatter you and what won't.

If you have a long thin face, then avoid wearing your hair long and straight with a centre parting. This will create a very harsh 'curtain' effect. You need to shorten your face, so a fringe will look good. Adding volume around your face with layers or curls will also help to pad it out.

If you have a round face, then a fringe is the worst thing you can do. A fringeless bob with a side parting so that one side of your hair cuts diagonally across your face is very flattering. Alternatively, you could go for a shorter style that sweeps back at the sides to give the impression that you have cheek bones.

If you have a square jaw, you need to soften it, otherwise you can look a bit stern. A feathered fringe and soft layers all over will be very flattering. Or, wear your hair in longer layers, with wispy bits brushed on to the jaw.

If you have a heart-shaped face, you are in a fortunate position because most styles suit you. Still, some heart shapes often have pointy chins. Creating a bit of width around a pointy chin is a way of softening it, so a chin-length bob works very well.

2

HAIR TYPE

If you dream of having a sleek Jennifer Aniston do, only your hair is naturally frizzy, then it's time to wake up. The reality could be a nightmare of daily straightening and struggling with hair products. You need to work with your hair type rather than fighting against it. It's a battle you will always lose.

If you have fine hair, styles that require masses of curls or ones that have a lot of fullness to them are going to be difficult for you to achieve. You can use hot rollers or a lot of blow-drying, but the condition of your hair will suffer. Instead go for sleek styles that complement your hair's natural straightness and silkiness.

If you have curly/frizzy hair, then put all thought of having a swingy bob out of your mind. It's not going to happen, honey. Instead, capitalize on the volume you can achieve. You could tame the frizz into recognizable curls and go for a romantic Pre-Raphaelite look, or cut it short. The curl will make it easy to style.

If you have Afro hair, the good news is that it is very versatile. You can quite literally sculpt it into any shape you want. If you keep it curly, you can go really big with it, or relax it and try a smoother, sleeker look. About the only styles you can't

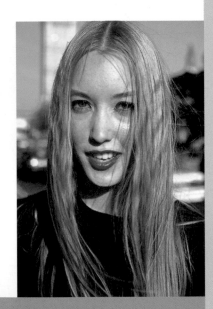

The cruellest style ever invented is the centre parting. Let's face it, when even a model looks a bit ropey, what hope is there for the rest of us?

Looking Good

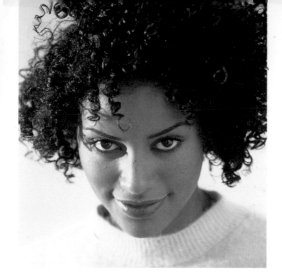

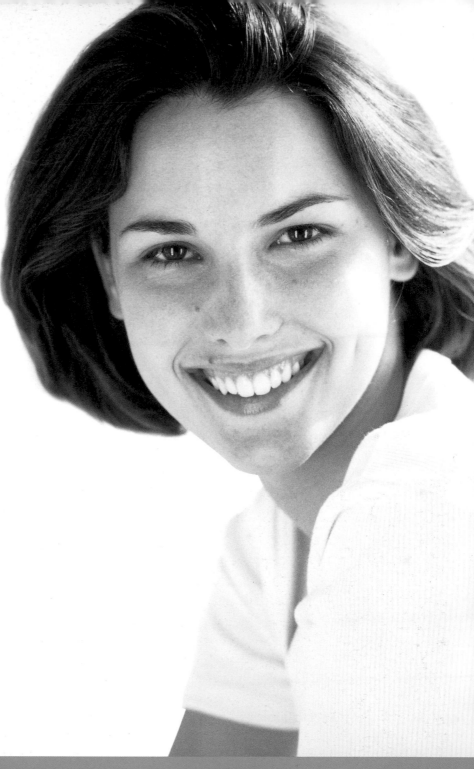

achieve are those that have lots of move-ment. Hair flicking or swinging is out.

If you have thick but straight hair, it can resemble a bush if you're not careful. Leaving it one length is the worst thing you can do. It will look far better if you either cut it very short, or layer it all over.

If you have thin hair, you are unlucky. This is the most difficult hair to work with. You will need to use lots of mousse and possibly rollers as well to give it some vol-ume. Another option is to colour it. A tint or highlights will thicken up each strand of hair, making the whole head look fuller.

3

HOW MUCH TIME YOU'RE WILLING TO SPEND STYLING IT

Many of us forget that the looks we see in magazines have often taken hours to achieve. How much time do you spend doing your own hair in the morning? Not that much, I reckon.

Think about how much time you will really be willing to spend on your hair each day. And be honest with yourself and your hairdresser. If you go for a look that requires serious styling and you can't be bothered, you're going to look an awful lot worse than if you'd gone for a simpler wash 'n' go style.

How much time do you have in the morning? If the answer is 'not a lot' and your locks are natu-rally curly (top left), forget about a sleek style (above).

Why can't I get my hair to look the way it did at the hair- dresser's?

There are two good reasons that your hair never looks as good as it did in the hair- dresser's. First off, the hairdresser can get right round the back of your head. Since you can't screw off your own head and walk round behind it, it is not really surprising that your efforts are less successful. Second, hairdressers spend years training so they can make our hair look good.

In a way, we've made a rod for our own backs. Our mothers and grandmothers often didn't even attempt to do their own hair at home. Up until the '60s, women went to a salon for a weekly shampoo and set. These days we don't want to carry around a concrete hairdo. We want to be able to wash our hair ourselves and that means styling it ourselves too...

'Mousse, gel or spritz, Madam?' The hair product explosion...

The number of products now on the market to help us achieve the salon look at home is huge – so huge, in fact, that it's difficult to know where to start. Lines range from cheap own-brand supermarket basics to 'designer' preparations. So what do you pick?

Designer shampoos: are they a rip-off?

It is tempting to dismiss all 'professional' hair lines as a waste of money. Certainly, some ranges launched by celebrity hair- dressers are heart-stoppingly expensive. And when you see their makers posing in their fabulous homes in *Hello!* you have to wonder what the mark-up is on this stuff.

When it comes to a basic shampoo, unless you're really, really picky about your hair (or you want a bathroom cabinet that looks drop dead chic) you're probably just as well buying a cheap one as an expensive one. All shampoo is basically detergent. The cheaper ones are usually more watered down detergent and may be a bit harsher.

If you are using a cheap shampoo how- ever, it won't remove all the gunk you collect on your hair. In fact, it may add some. Apart from grime and pollution, your hair will build up a residue from all the products (including shampoo) that you use on it. So, once a month it's a good idea to use a purifying shampoo. Neutrogena shampoo is one of the best. It is expensive, but you need only a little and you are using it only once a month.

Where 'designer' lines come into their own is in the add-on products – the curl relaxers, the silicon serums, the deep condi- tioners. Professional lines drive the whole hair product industry forward. Because they are expensive, they can afford to do research and development and come up with new things. Only once these have proved suc- cessful do cheaper lines become available.

All these new ideas can be confusing, however. So how do you know what to use?

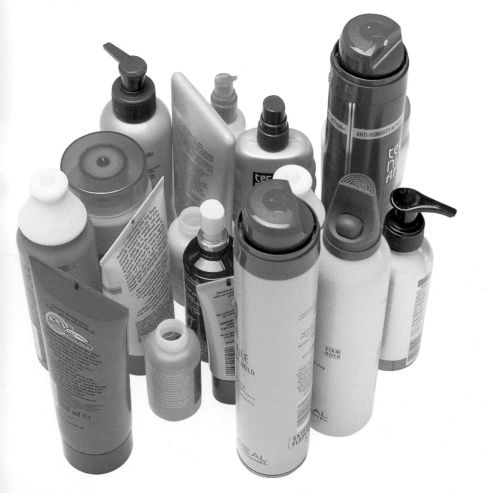

Gels

Gels were one of the first hair products to come on to the market in the '80s. They provide hold, but can make the hair feel sticky and even look a bit flaky.

Correct application: take a pound coin-sized blob of gel in your hand and smooth it through wet or dry hair. Comb through thoroughly. If your hair is wet, blow-dry it.

Mousses

The second most popular holding medium, mousses also provide volume, but they can be sticky and dull shine.

Correct application: spray a golf ball-sized blob into the bristle side of a flat brush. Use more if you have longer hair. Brush through wet hair. Make sure you get the same amount on the roots as you do at the ends. The reason why it's a good idea to use a brush is that with your hands, application can be a bit haphazard. Style and dry in the normal way.

Spritzing sprays

The successor to gels and mousses, spritzing sprays don't give a sticky feeling but hold well. They won't give you much volume

Correct application: spray directly on to a section of wet hair. It dries quickly, so you only want to apply it to the bit of hair you are drying.

Hair spray

The old favourite, it gives great hold, but no volume and can 'mat' the hair together.

Correct application: unlike spritzing sprays, hair spray can be used only on dry hair. Style as required, then spray directly on to the area you want held.

Serums

These protect the hair from heat damage caused by blow-drying and also improve shine. However, they don't give very much volume.

Correct application: put a tiny amount in the palm of your hand and rub over the wet ends of your hair. Style as normal.

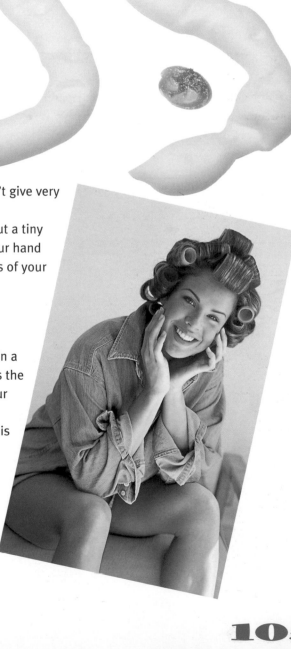

Laminators

No, you won't find these in a stationers. Laminators, as the name suggests, make your hair more shiny.

Correct application: this depends on the type of laminator being used. With a gel, you squeeze a tiny amount from the tube and smooth it on. With a spray, apply it to dry hair after you have styled it.

I want root lift and I want it now

There are three ways to get it. The first is to tip your head upside down when you are blow-drying your hair. This works but can cause static electricity. The second way is to use hot rollers. Easy to do, but these can cause long-term damage to your hair if you use them every day.

The third and most tricky way is to use a comb and hairdryer. Wash and towel dry your hair. Comb it through. Then, working in small sections, part the hair. Put the comb in at the root of a clump of hair, lift the hair and fold the comb over, embedding the teeth of the comb back into the other side of the clump. What you are doing is sort of pleating the root of the hair. Dry with a hairdryer. If it has a cold setting on it, blast the roots with cold air before moving on to the next section. Once all the roots are dry, you style the rest of your hair.

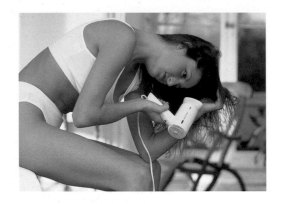

Clips, bows, etc.

I am not a big fan of hair accessories. Memories of Fergie and her horrible helicopter hair clips come to mind. In my view, hair accessories are the female version of novelty boxer shorts for men. The person who wears either is as good as saying, 'I'm mad, I am,' and I want to back away from them very quickly. That said, if you want to adorn yourself with accessories, keep them as simple as possible.

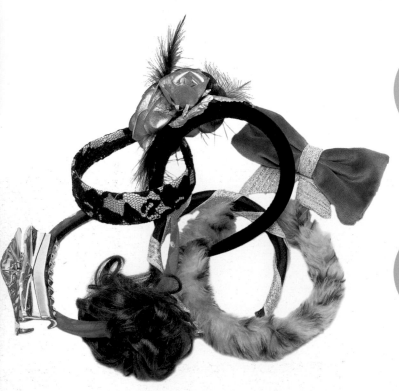

HAIR ACCESSORY HORRORS

wide velvet Alice bands

wide patterned Alice bands

wide patterned Alice bands with bows, ribbons, pearls or diamanté on

HAIR ACCESSORIES YOU CAN GET AWAY WITH

narrow gold or silver metal hair bands

diamanté clips

tortoiseshell combs

Other accessories are a bit of a grey area. The jury's still out on squidgies. They are not remotely fashionable, but where would we be without them? A bit like the average man, really.

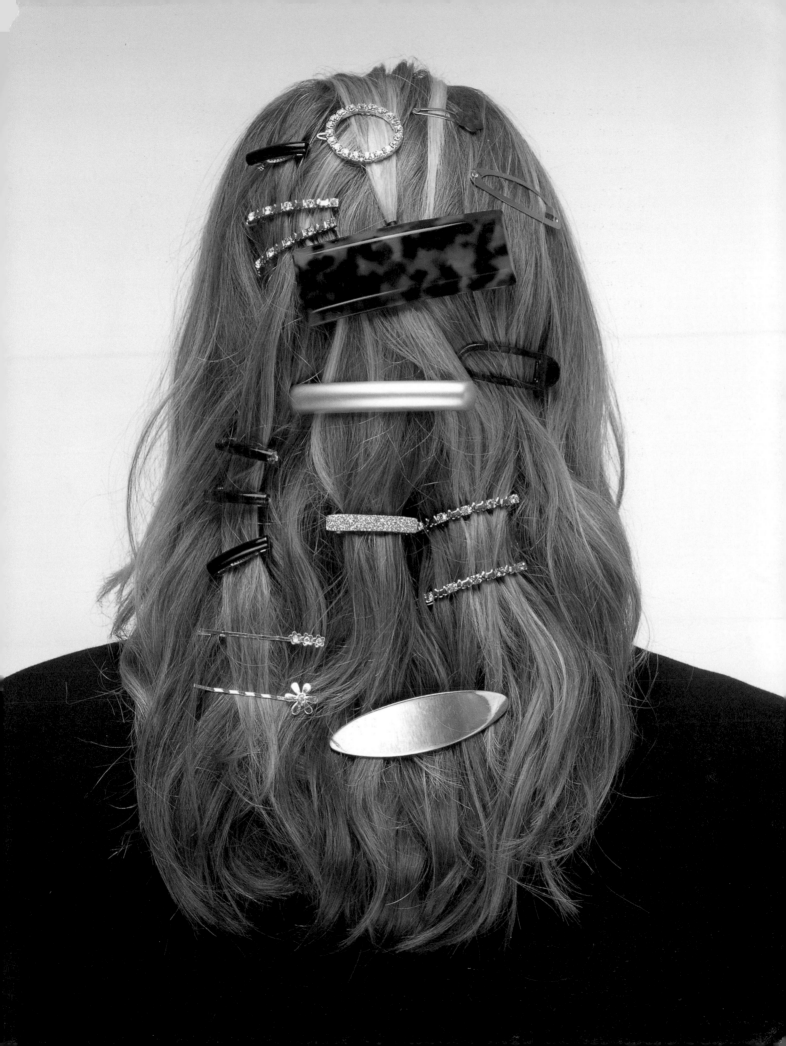

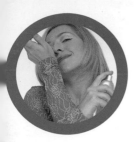

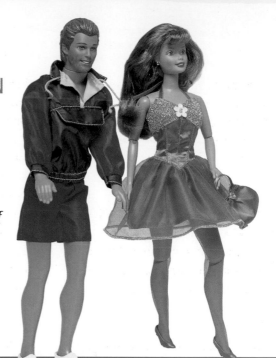

You know how it is. You start off in your teens looking for the perfect man. In your twenties, you've downshifted to a search for a semi-perfect male.

You're looking good,
but he still looks like a
dog's breakfast

By the time you've hit thirty, you'll take basically anything so long as he's:

1 single
2 heterosexual
3 got all his bits

If he's got a naff wardrobe, well, that's the least of your worries. It's his personality that matters, you tell yourself. His sparkling wit, stunning repartee, the fact that he takes the rubbish out and knows how to fix the car when it breaks down, these are the qualities that draw you to him. And if he does happen to wear jackets with patches on the elbows, knitted tank tops and shirts covered in lurid checks, frankly, you're not that shallow. Except you keep looking at those jackets and the knitwear and the shirts and you really hate yourself, but YOU HATE THEM!

I went out with a man a few years ago who was ideal in every respect. He was bright, funny and nice to me. He even cooked me dinner. He ran his own company, so he could also afford to take me out occasionally. The night we met, I set light to my hair by accident – wine bars with candles in bottles on tables should be banned – and he was very sweet about that. The problem was his clothes.

On our first date he wore a baggy navy jumper, beige cords and shoes like Cornish pasties. He wore this horrible outfit on the second and the third date too. By date five, I was at the end of my tether. While he cooked dinner, I nipped upstairs and had a look in his wardrobe. He had five of those jumpers, five pairs of those trousers, even five pairs of those shoes. Up to that moment, I had consoled myself with the thought that over time

I might be able to wean him away from his cords, etc. Now I realized it would take me years. Could I wait that long? Actually, no. We parted shortly after and I have to admit that the Cornish pasty shoes were a factor.

Oh no! I'm dating a fashion phobic

If you find yourself going out with or even married to someone who has no taste in clothes, you have three choices:

1 Ditch him immediately.
2 Sit him down and have a serious talk with him.
3 Restyle him by stealth.

The first is a bit too drastic for most. Divorce on the grounds of unreasonable knitwear is not yet, I think, allowable in this country. The second option is no less difficult, however. It is amazing how a man will dig his heels in if you tell him everything in his wardrobe is disgusting. In a pointless effort to assert his masculinity, he will deliberately put on the article you have confessed to hate. Either that, or he may even go out and buy more versions of it.

This leaves us with the stealth option. A bit underhand perhaps, but remember, it's for his own good. You will be much better disposed towards him if he doesn't embarrass you in front of your friends by wearing horrible clothes.

How to give him a make-over without him noticing

STEP ONE

The first step is get rid of a few items immediately. These are the things that make you feel positively queasy. There are various ways to do this. Clothing can be 'accidentally' ruined in the wash. A red sock slipped in with his favourite cream top, or a cardi he likes mistakenly put on boil wash, that sort of thing.

Alternatively, if the garment you loathe is a non-washable item, you can offer to take it to the dry cleaner. Chuck it in a bin on your way and then a week later claim that the dry cleaning machine chewed it up. Take it to a dry cleaner you don't normally use though, so you can make a big thing of boycotting it after such 'appalling' service without inconveniencing yourself too much.

Or why not make him do the work for you? Suggest he wears the offending item out to dinner. A curry is a good choice. Go to the ladies and on the way back bash into him by mistake. You need to time your sudden clumsiness at the exact moment a forkful of curry is in transit from plate to mouth. Then he'll spill it all down the front of the garment you hate. Again, offer to wash it for him and claim not to be able to get the curry out.

STEP TWO

This is where you replace items that might have been 'lost' or 'damaged' with things you prefer. Take him shopping and, out of the goodness of your heart, offer to buy him things. Make sure you take only him to shops you like, and even case them first to make sure there is nothing awful that his eye might alight upon.

When you are in the shop, send him into the changing room and have a quiet word with the assistant. Most assistants know that if a couple are shopping together, it's the woman who's in charge. So if you ask them nicely, they are sure to point your other half in the direction you want him to go.

A variation on this approach is to buy him clothes as presents for Christmas and birthdays. The good thing about doing this is that you don't have to go through the charade of being seen to listen to his opinion. You just buy what you want him to wear, no arguments.

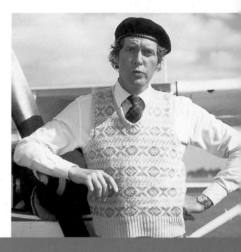

Frank Spencer, aka Tank-Top Man

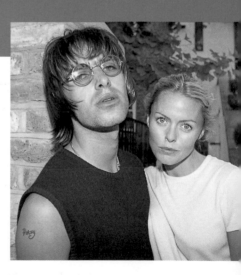

Nice tee-shirt, shame about the boyfriend. Patsy is let down by Liam.

Step three

This is where you really grasp the nettle. Offer to give his wardrobe a spring clean. Say you're doing yours or there is a car boot sale at the local school or something. If he isn't keen, you may have to move house to persuade him a sort-out is essential. Depending on how bad his clothes are, changing your address might be the lesser of two evils.

I once re-organized my partner's wardrobe while he was out. To be fair, he had asked me to have a sort-out of his shirts. I filled six dustbin bags with shirts, jumpers, trousers, even suits, coats and shoes. I took them all immediately to Oxfam. He was not happy when he got home. But, hey, he got over it.

You don't have to be that drastic. It depends on how strong your relationship is. I suggest you wait until at least the third date before you start emptying his cupboards. And, if you do manage to have a clear-out, make sure you send the stuff to a charity shop a fair distance away or he'll go and get it all back again. My sister's husband did that.

Above: Gazza proving why a man should never be allowed to shop on his own.

Step four

This is optional and is in fact more a revenge tactic than a resettling one. You have a little bonfire of the garments you hate. It is very cathartic, but there is no going back. I have a girlfriend who thought her boyfriend had been unfaithful. She barbecued his prize Man U shirt. When she found out he hadn't played away, she was mortified but kept quiet. He asked what had happened to his shirt for months.

So what is the fashionable man wearing this year?

If you have managed to clear out the really horrible stuff from his wardrobe, what do you replace it with? Fortunately, menswear tends to change at a slower pace than womenswear does. So if you buy a few classics, they should last him a while.

This is your shopping list:

CASUAL

2 pairs jeans – black and blue. If in doubt, Levi 501s

1 pair beige cotton chinos

1 pair beige cotton walking shorts

2 pairs jogging bottoms – black and grey

6 tee-shirts – 2 white, 2 black, 2 grey

3 sweatshirts – white, grey, black

4 white cotton casual long-sleeved shirts – 2 white, 2 blue

3 plain cotton jumpers – black, grey, navy

2 cotton bomber jackets, 1 beige, one black

1 pair leather loafers/deck shoes

1 pair trainers

This is a very restricted list, colourwise, but best not to confuse him.

WORK

3 single-breasted suits – black, navy, dark grey

5 cotton shirts – 3 white, 2 blue

6 ties – 2 with a navy ground, 2 black, 2 grey

1 black belt

2 pairs black lace-up shoes

6 pairs socks - 2 black, 2 navy, 2 grey

1 beige mac

You, or he, don't have to spend an enormous amount of money on this revamp, but make sure he has his suits dry cleaned regularly. It is amazing how many men will wear a suit until it can stand up on its own.

A man and his hair – a very special relationship

If you've ever tried to get a man to change his hair, you'll know that it is almost impossible. Men are very touchy about their hair – even if they're not losing it. If they are going thin on top, just bringing up the subject will have him reaching for the paracetamol.

For those chaps who are thinning a bit, the only choice is to keep it short. Better to brazen it out than do a Bobby Charlton. However, for many men, hair equals their sex appeal. A whole generation – those over 45 – equates hair that passes their collar at back as a major anti-establishment statement. Short of creeping up behind him with some clippers when he is sleeping, you will not get him to cut it.

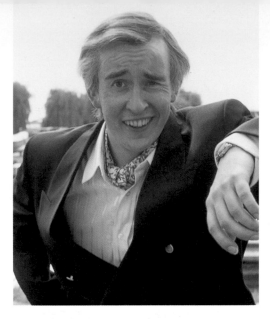

Television's favourite blazer and slacks man: Alan Partridge demonstrates the 'brush across'.

Medallions and all that

Jewellery on a man is almost invariably dreadful. Apart from a wedding ring and a decent watch, it should be eschewed. Tie pins and necklaces worn over ties are an absolute no-no.

There are some men who won't be told, of course. My Cornish pasty bloke was a case in point. So before you waste too much energy, here's how to spot a lost cause at a glance.

1
LEATHER JACKET MAN
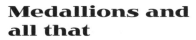

He is probably in middle age, if not in the middle of a mid-life crisis. He wears his leather jacket stretched over a beer belly. He may or may not drive a sports car. Cowboy boots will lurk somewhere in his wardrobe. It may be a phase, but there will be no shifting him out of it.

2
SHELLSUIT MAN
He is interested only in comfort. Trying to get him to wear anything other than baggy polyester will be impossible. He will probably never have put on a pair of proper shoes. If you can get him to change his tee-shirt on a regular basis, quit while you're ahead.

3
BLAZER AND SLACKS MAN
Seen at Rotary Club functions, this chap thinks he's dapper. He is a firm believer in the benefits of clothes brushes and polishing his shoes. He probably wears a cravat in bed. Steer well clear.

4
HEAVY METAL MAN
He will have long hair and tight jeans and even tighter tee-shirts. Everything will be black, slightly faded. For him, his rock look is a sign of teenage rebellion. Point out he's no longer a teenager and he'll get into a strop. Leave him in peace with his air guitar.

P.S.

Any men reading this chapter might think it a tad sexist, but I make no apologies. However, if your partner is now bristling with indignation at the suggestion that he cannot be trusted to buy his own clothes, I have one last tip – the same as I'd give those whose enjoyment of the *Looking Good* programme is interrupted by a whingey male: tell him to shove off and read a car magazine. We girls deserve a bit of territory of our own, don't we?

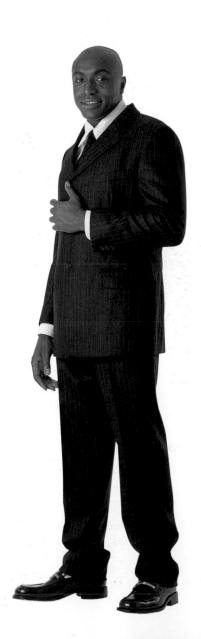

This book is published to accompany the BBC TV series *Looking Good*.

Series Producer: Jeanine Josman

Published by BBC Worldwide Ltd, Woodlands, 80 Wood Lane, London W12 0TT

First published in 1999

Specially commissioned photography (for jacket and inside the book) by Ray Moller,
© BBC Books, 1999. Special photography styled by Fleur Britten.
For other photography credits, please see below.

ISBN 0 563 38486 7

Commissioning Editor: Viv Bowler
Art Director/Book Designer: Lisa Pettibone
Cover Design: DW Design
Project Editor: Lara Speicher
Picture Researcher: Miriam Hyman
Printed and bound in France by Imprimerie Pollina s.a.
Colour separations by Radstock Reproductions Ltd, Midsomer Norton

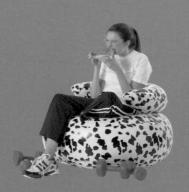

BBC Books would like to thank the following for providing photographs and for permission to reproduce copyright material. While every effort has been made to trace and acknowledge all copyright holders, we would like to apologize should there have been any errors or omissions.

l (left), r (right), m (middle), t (top), b (bottom).

Ace pages 16t (Jigsaw), 26r (Colin Thomas), 28b (Michael Melia), 37t Benelux Press, 37br (Alex Bruce), 52b (Graham Tucker), 75m (Colin Thomas); **The Advertising Archives** 82b, 88b; **Attard** 34tr, 94, 95r; © **BBC** 12tr, 67b, 69l, 69m, 109t, 111t; **Berkertex Brides** 74; **Big Pictures** 86r; **Camera Press** 98 (Denzil McNeelance), 100b (Chris Ashford), 102t (Theodre Wood); **Jimmy Choo** 58tr; **Corbis/UPI** 33r; **Formes (UK) Ltd** 78tr, 79b, 80b, 81; **Ronald Grant Archives** 29b, 33b, 34bl; **Robert Harding Picture Library** 16b, 31tl, 31tr, 31b, 36l, 39b, 40b, 41t, 51t, 55, 61m, 62l, 63b, 84, 85t, 89r, 92, 93tl, 93tr, 99t, 100tr; **The Image Bank** 19bl, 91m, 93bl, 93br, 105b; **Images** 23, 28t, 29t, 32, 39t, 53t, 63mr, 79t, 89l; **Marks and Spencer** 45t, 64b, 65m; **Chris Moore Photography** 52tr, 65b, 83t, 90; **Muji** 11t; **Next** 24, 31m, 33tl, 44, 45b, 47b, 57t, 62m, 63ml; **PA News** 11b; **Pictor International** 72b, 102b, 103l; **PolyGram/Pictorial Press** 75t; **Janet Reger** 38tl, 38b; **Rex Features** 17t, 19t, 27t, 41b, 43r, 47t, 53b, 58br, 61t, 62r, 63m, 67t, 69b, 70r, 71, 76, 77, 80t, 109b, 110t; **The Stock Market Photo Agency UK** 12b, 13, 15b, 42, 43l, 51b, 91l; **Tony Stone Images** s 8b (Nancy Honey), 9t (Donna Day), 17b (David Hanover), 19br (Eric Larrayadieu), 20t (Susan Werner), 21 (Bernard Pesce), 22b (David Stewart), 46b (Joe Polollio), 57b (Christopher Bissell), 60t (Timothy Shonnard), 64t (Nick Dolding), 72tr (Donna Day), 82tr (Bob Thomas), 99b (Jerome Tisne), 101 (James Darrell), 103r (Jerome Tisne), 106t (James Darrell); **Virgin Brides** 73b, 75r; **Wealth of the Nations** 25; **Wonderbra/Playtex** 35.

All remaining photographs by Ray Moller © BBC Books, 1999
We would like to thank the following for kindly supplying their products for the special photography:

Watches **Swatch** page 8tl; Drawer dividers **The Holding Company** 10ml; Scarves **Gordana** 12tl; Cardie on hanger **Miss Selfridge**, top **River Island** 15t; Trying on top from **'Y'** 18; Control garment **Marks and Spencer** 22tr; Glasses and boa from **Mikey** 26l; Dress **Hobbs**, shoes **Jimmy Choo** 30; **Gossard Wonderbra** 36r; Phone **Swatch** 46tl; Pinstripe suit and shoes **Hobbs** 49l; Tights **Sock Shop** 54; Tights **Pretty Polly** and **Aristoc** 56; Lowri holds shoes **Faith** 58tl; Trainers **Buffalo** 59t; Shoes **Faith** 59b; Shoes **Debenhams, Barratts, Faith, Ravel, Jimmy Choo** and **River Island** 60-61; Shoes **Barratts** 65tl; Long grey dress **Evans**, mannequins's skirt and top **Nicole Farhi**, mannequin **Mannequin World Visuals** 66r; Suit **Hobbs**, jewellery **Agatna** 68; Coat and top **Long Tall Sally**, boots **Hobbs**, skirt **LTS** 70l; Hat **The Hat Shop** 73t; Swimsuit **Jantzen** 83b; Sarongs **Gottex** 85b and 86l; Make-up **Spectacular, Rimmel, Chanel** and **L'Oreal** 88tr; Brushes **The Body Shop** and **Shu Vemura** 95l; Hair products **L'Oreal** and **The Body Shop** 104; Hair accessories **Accessorize** and **Agatna** 107; Trousers **Eddie Baner**, shirt **Savane**, coat **Next**, shoes **Nicole Farhi** 110b; Suit, shirt and tie **Reiss**, shoes **Boss** 111b.

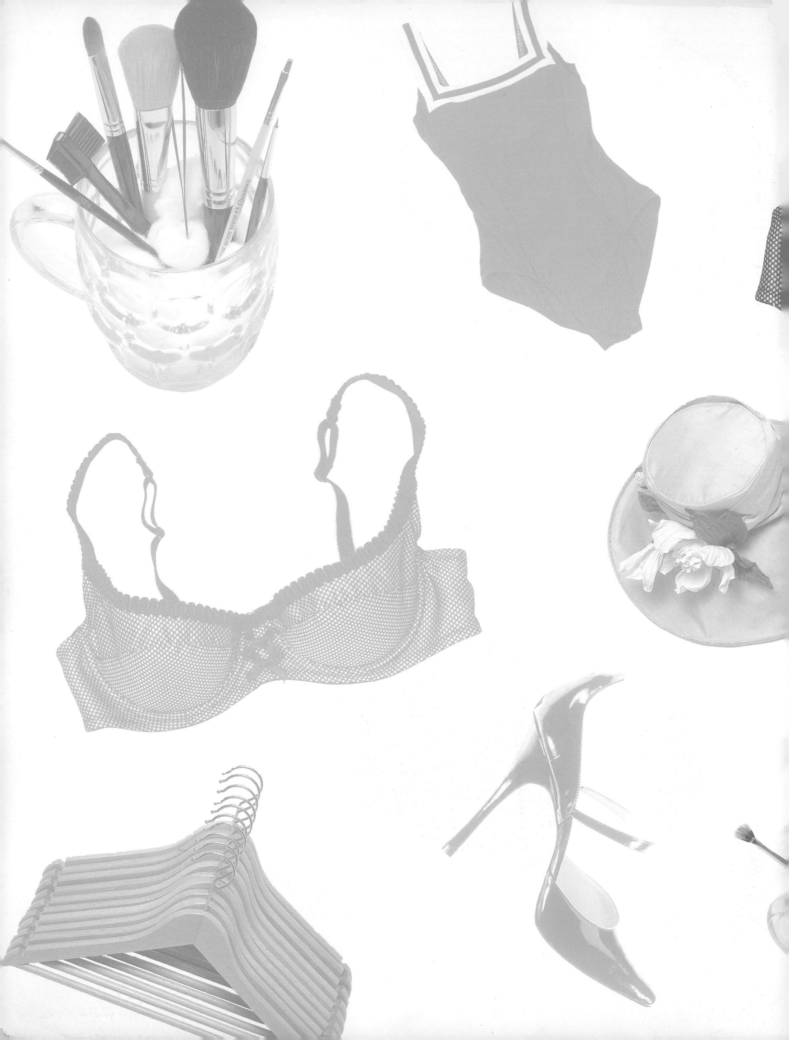

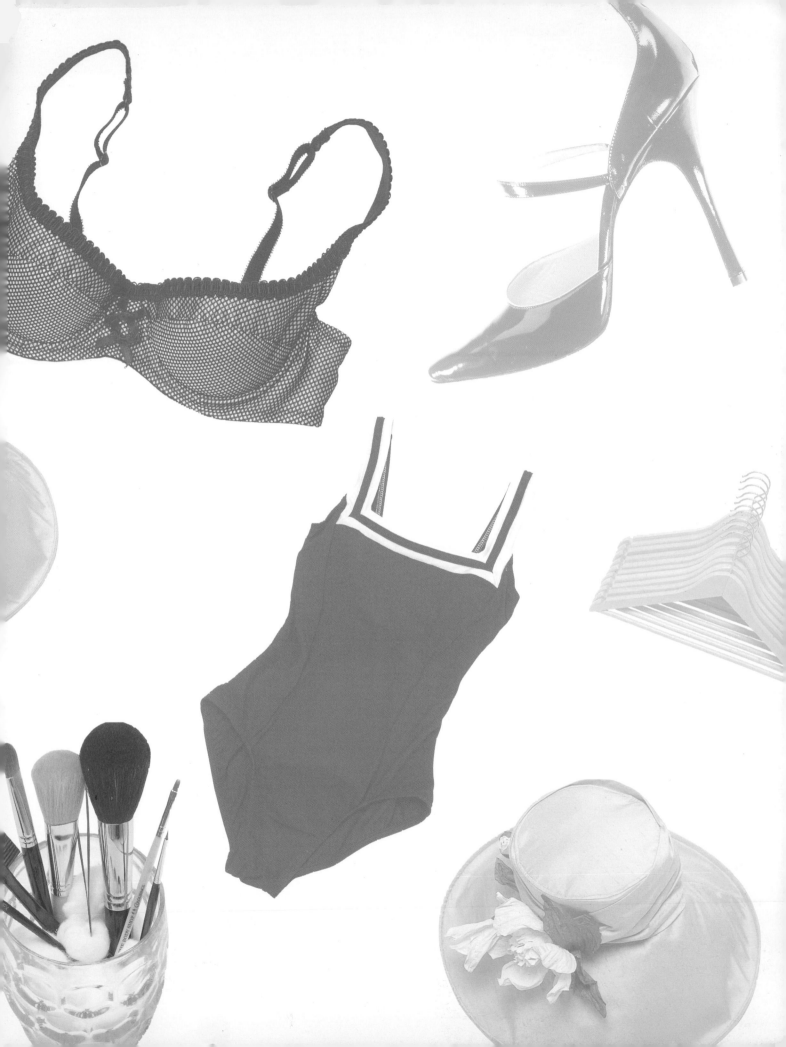

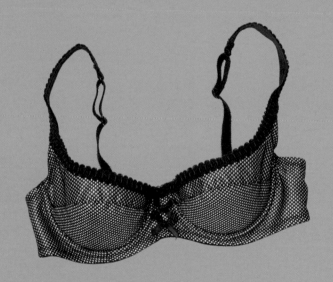